STARVING IN SEARCH OF ME

**A Coming-of-Age Story
of Overcoming an Eating Disorder
and Finding Self-Acceptance**

by
MARISSA LAROCCA

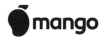

Published by Mango Publishing Group, a division of Mango Media Inc.

Cover Design: Marissa LaRocca and Morgane Leoni
Layout & Design: Morgane Leoni

For permission requests, please contact the publisher at:
Mango Publishing Group
2850 Douglas Road, 3rd Floor
Coral Gables, FL 33134 U.S.A.
info@mango.bz

For special orders, quantity sales, course adoptions and corporate sales, please email the publisher at sales@mango.bz. For trade and wholesale sales, please contact Ingram Publisher Services at customer.service@ingramcontent.com or +1.800.509.4887.

Starving in Search of Me: A Coming-of-Age Story of Overcoming an Eating Disorder and Finding Self-Acceptance

Library of Congress Cataloging
ISBN: (p) 978-1-63353-712-5, (e) 978-1-63353-713-2
Library of Congress Control Number: 2017916449
BISAC SEL014000 SELF-HELP / Eating Disorders & Body Image

Printed in the United States of America

To my former self, and to those currently struggling to find comfort in their bodies, in the world.

Table of Content

Foreword

I first met Marissa about ten years ago. I happened to be dating her twin sister Kristy at the time. We were all queer in our early twenties, each of us on an existential quest to understand ourselves in a world that was only beginning to unfold.

Marissa had an eating disorder back then. The first time I came to understand the severity of it was one Christmas when I accompanied Kristy and Marissa's family to their Aunt and Uncle's house. We all ate a good amount of food—first an array of appetizers, then an array of dinner options, and a colorful array of desserts. Soon after, I found Marissa locked in the bathroom in the basement and she confided in me that she was struggling with what she had consumed. I was able to identify because I'd gone through an eating disorder myself just a couple of years prior and was still very familiar with the urges. From then on it was something we would talk about every now and then, whenever we found ourselves on someone's stoop smoking a cigarette after a few drinks.

Another memory comes to mind simply because there's irony in it—I was lying on the beach with Kristy, reading *The Power of Now* by Eckhart Tolle. Kristy and

I were deeply interested in Buddhist philosophy. In the process of defining ourselves, and our relationship, we were drawn to the lessons presented by this book: *All life is a series of present moments; Pain is the result of resisting things we cannot change; The ego is a powerful weapon that need not limit or define us—we can free ourselves from suffering by cultivating self-awareness and not judging our thoughts.*

On this particular day, we invited Marissa to sit with us to read and watch the ocean but, instead, Marissa was revved up in her running shorts and sneakers, ready to burn calories by running laps around the beach. The irony was that Kristy and I were reading a book about surrendering to the present moment and Marissa was running, quite literally, away from it. She was running away from herself in the way so many young women do.

I was just nine years old when I first considered the relationship between food and my body. I had a ballet teacher pinch my love handle fat and say, "Don't go telling your parents I called you fat." By the age of eleven or twelve, there were weeks when all I'd eat were peanut butter and jelly sandwiches. And into my teen years, I was primarily anorexic. I calculated every calorie that went into my body, consuming under five hundred calories some days. Of course, my dance teachers all praised my petite frame. I got cast in every lead role in every ballet show we put on. And the more attention I got, the more it reinforced this notion that starving myself was *good*. Starving myself was my ticket to opportunities and admiration I would not have otherwise received. Restricting my diet to such an extreme was difficult to keep up with, considering the amount of dancing I was doing, so I'd have "binge days," which left me feeling indescribably horrible. I never purged; I just couldn't bring myself to do that. But I definitely had days where I danced for four hours, ate very little, and completed an hour of Tae Bo before bed.

In a recent conversation, Marissa asked me, "Do you consider yourself fully healed from your eating disorder?" In my response I said, "I don't think I can consider myself healed unless I considered myself broken before, and I never considered myself broken." Mental disorders don't define people or their state of being. They are just experiences we have along our journeys to learning who we are. Do I allow food to control me now? No. Do I starve myself? Definitely not; I consider nourishing my body to be one of my highest priorities. So, the simple answer would be, "Yes, I consider myself healed." I consider myself happy and healthy. But do I still have moments? Days? Thoughts? Yes, of course. I relate my recovery to that of any addict. You can be an alcoholic and sober for years, but you're still an alcoholic. The difference is you've learned to become stronger than your thoughts and get in touch with something deeper in yourself, or something bigger than you, which gives you a perspective that enables you to make healthier decisions for your own well-being. This is the closest thing to "healed" that I think I can be: focused on self-love and willing to surrender to one day at a time.

As a YouTube vlogger, plant-based advocate, and LGBTQ activist, I've had the privilege of touching the lives of hundreds of thousands of people around the world. I receive hundreds of messages daily, mostly from girls thanking me for helping them in big or small ways just by being ME and sharing what I've been through. I say this in my videos constantly, but if I could send one message to young people today, it would be this: YOU ARE WORTHY. I truly believe in my heart that every single human being on this planet has purpose and massive potential, and too often it goes unrealized. Since "recovering" from my own addictions, I am able to see self-harm and self-hate as ways in which the negative energy in the world (or the dark sides within us) try to bring us down and shut off our light so we can't shine. I say, be your own kind of beautiful. Speak out. Share who you really are. Prove society wrong.

I think *Starving in Search of Me* is a significant work of honesty that is going to provide company and hope to many who are struggling with the weight of a world that isn't always easy to stand out in. Now more than ever before, I think that young people need courageous voices like Marissa's to guide and reassure them that what makes them different is what makes them beautiful. And what makes us suffer makes us human—we are all connected to one another through shared experiences of triumph, failure, and vulnerability.

If you've ever struggled with an eating disorder, or any other form of self-harm or addiction, I am confident that what you are about to witness in the coming pages will resonate and gracefully navigate you toward hope, meaning, and light. In my opinion, Marissa has accomplished something pretty substantial here—she's found a way to articulate in words the intangible depths of an experience that is hers, and all of ours.

ABOUT KATE[1]

Also known as Kate Fruit Flowers, Kate is a popular influencer on YouTube, notable for LGBTQ and vegan-friendly content which garnered her 200,000 subscribers. She began studying the effects of a holistic plant-based approach in 2009.

1. Famous Birthdays. "Kate Flowers." https://www.famousbirthdays.com/people/kate-flowers.html (accessed 2017).

Introduction

-

"There is no greater agony than bearing an untold story inside you."
–Maya Angelou

-

Dear Reader,

I remember the day I decided to attempt writing about my experiences with an eating disorder. It was my senior year of college, and I sat before a blank Word document in the campus library with the cursor blinking for at least thirty minutes before a single word came to mind. I had become so detached from my emotions at that point that giving a voice to the fragile, feeling parts of myself felt foreign, even impossible. But after years of enduring a very intense, very private battle with food and exercise, and knowing I was on the road to recovery, I felt I had something meaningful to say. I had traveled to places few people have gone and I had seen things few people have seen. I was convinced I might write the next *New York Times* bestseller, if only I could get a single sentence onto paper.

It's been nine years since that day, and in that time, I've felt an ongoing urgency to "figure myself out." That is, to peel back the complicated layers and understand what led me to struggle with this addiction in the first place. Was it a cry for help? If so, what kind of help was I seeking? Was it an experiment? If so, what was I hoping to gain by challenging my physical limits? Was it a spiritual quest? If yes, then what inspired me to want to expand beyond the physical world and connect with something greater? Sure, I've always felt "different." But I come from a good family and a good home. In the eyes of any onlooker, I have not suffered any real hardships in my life. Yet what hijacked my reality was something so dark and so powerful, something all-encompassing that swallowed me whole.

The interesting thing I've come to realize in the process of reflecting and writing about my eating disorder is that what appeared to be a food disorder really had nothing to do with food at all. My addiction was the thing I used to distract me from my pain. It was a coping mechanism that enabled me to avoid dealing with my real issues—an undeveloped sense of self, social anxiety, and confusion around my sexuality, among other identity roadblocks. I was not yet equipped with the tools to nurture myself, or the courage to make my needs known to others, and so I clung to very deliberate behaviors that had predictable outcomes…like starving myself.

As more and more of this developed in my awareness, I began to consider the relationship between my eating disorder and the reoccurring feelings of my adolescence—feeling like I didn't fit in, feeling like I couldn't stand up for myself, and feeling like I didn't always deserve to take up space in the world. All the while I was dodging calories, purging, and compulsively exercising, I was *actually* just trying to protect myself from a reality that felt dangerous and unsafe.

This was a pretty big realization for me, in that it prompted me to think more openly about addiction and mental illness as a whole. I began to wonder: to what extent are disorders actually "disorders," and to what extent are they doorways to helping us understand the truth about our lives? Many people engage in self-deprecating or even masochistic behaviors to help them cope with an underlying challenge at some point in their existence. Are all of these people sick? Or can we empower them instead and say they simply haven't yet accessed the parts of themselves that hold the key to their healing? Perhaps at the root of all addiction is the refusal to acknowledge or permit certain feelings—feelings that, if witnessed, have the power to free their sufferers. Perhaps the suffering is even *part* of the journey to healing.

Then there's society and the rest of the world to consider. While it's definitely not my prerogative to defend eating disorders or other acts of self-harm, I do believe their prevalence in our modern world is an epidemic that must be compassionately examined. Though commonly experienced in isolation, such "disorders" represent a collective yearning for connection, acceptance, and emotional nourishment among generations that are starving for many things. Simply organizing sufferers of anorexia, bulimia, and other issues into their respective boxes based on an exhibited list of symptoms and treating them accordingly is not enough to heal them. We need to dig deeper. We need to ask, "Who are the human beings beneath these labels? And what are they *really* hungry for?"

The experience of writing this book has been both therapeutic and agonizing. In trying to untangle what began as a heavy, abstract knot of thoughts and emotions, I've learned quite a few things about myself—things that have given me a clearer direction not only in writing this book, but in living my life. In addition to having some meaningful things to share with others, it turns out that I also had a lot to uncover for myself and a lot of growing to do. I appreciate you taking the time to witness the parts of this journey I've managed to transcribe.

At thirty-one years old, I'm happy to say I no longer struggle with an eating disorder of any kind. While I admit I'm a work in progress like anyone else, I've developed a sense of awareness, compassion, and appreciation for myself that makes it feel impossible now for me to disparage myself in any way. In discovering who I am and what I need to feel sane in the world, I've opened myself up to a reality where I'm able to be more trusting and forgiving toward myself and others. I recognize now that it's my own responsibility to take care of myself, and with the realization of this responsibility comes a great deal of power.

In the following pages, I'll share with you everything I've come to understand about my hunger and all of its implications. While this book might be most relevant to those who have experienced or are currently experiencing an eating disorder, I think it will make a good companion for anyone who's struggled with identity, sexuality, or an addiction of any kind. Regardless of who you are and where you're coming from, I am thankful for the opportunity to reach you.

Marissa

PART 1:
WHAT'S EATING THE WALLFLOWER

Chapter 1
WHY ARE YOU SO QUIET?

-

In this first section, I'll share with you my personal story with as much gritty emotional truth as I can. I'll tell you about how I felt like an outcast throughout my school years due to being painfully introverted, how I related to my family, how I felt plagued with fear and confusion around my sexuality beginning around puberty, and how I struggled to transition from adolescence into adulthood with only a frighteningly subtle sense of who I was and what I needed to be happy.

EARLY STRUGGLES WITH SOCIAL ANXIETY AND FITTING IN

To this day, I'm not sure there's anything more terrifying than entering the cafeteria alone on the first day of school. For an eternal moment, you hover in the entranceway, watching everyone take a seat as if choreographed, as if summer was just another day gone by and no one's kinships have skipped a beat. Then the bell rings with a frantic shrill, and soon enough you're the only one left standing. What do you do? Your backpack weighs on your adolescent shoulders, heavy with too many textbooks. It's too late to be inconspicuous. You have to make a decision. Now really, what *do* you do?

Both literally and metaphorically, I've never really known where to sit. So I spent many of my elementary and high school lunch periods hiding out in a stall in the girls' bathroom, discreetly peeling the aluminum foil off my peanut butter and jelly sandwich, hoping to God no one would notice my feet under the door.

From the time I was very young, I sensed there was something different about me. I was first exposed to people my age at a Catholic elementary school, and it didn't come naturally to me to reach out of my comfort zone and make friends. I was highly observant, perceptive, and painfully shy. While the other kids goofed off during recess and competed for attention during gym class, I sat watching them, harboring this feeling that there were infinite universes between me and other human beings. A wallflower by nature, I did the best I could to conceal my nerves and blend in. But I very quickly learned that keeping to myself was a widely unacceptable manner of existing.

"Why are you so quiet?" my classmates would ask me, interrupting the concentrated effort I put into trying to make myself invisible.

"I don't know," I'd reply with a bashful grin and eyes that begged them to leave me alone. Then I'd return to my default personality—well behaved and petrified. Eventually, through the years, my classmates stopped asking questions, and I was just the quiet girl in class who did all her homework and rarely raised her hand.

I remember getting on the school bus, always choosing the third or fourth seat. The middle of the bus, slightly favoring the front, felt safest to me. Of course, the back of the bus was reserved for the cooler kids, the rowdy troublemakers and the itchy little perverts. And the first two rows were for those with some quality about them considered by the cooler kids to be a drastic impediment—the boy with the stutter, the girl with the retainer that wrapped around her whole head. So by choosing the middle, I made a commitment to my place within the unspoken social hierarchy—I wasn't cool, but I wasn't a "loser" either. I was just there, lost beneath the hum of the school bus engine and the indistinct chatter, wanting to draw as little attention to myself as possible.

My parents were never religious people. I'm pretty sure they sent my sister and I to Catholic school thinking that we'd get a better education than in public school, and we'd be safer. And that may have been true. But I do wonder to what extent I may have been negatively impacted by the years of seeing Jesus nailed to a cross, with the nuns and priests reinforcing this as the ultimate symbol of sacrifice. Throughout my formative years, when my mind was most impressionable, I was taught that sinning is *bad*; people who sin burn forever in hell. God was a powerful man in the sky and I was a little girl on the ground being evaluated for the "goodness" or "badness" of my every decision. Then they told me I was already made of sin for being a human being because Adam and Eve ate an apple that God told them not to eat. And so every morning after the first school bell, my entire class had to recite the Our Father prayer in unison. "Lead us not into temptation, but deliver us from evil. Amen."

In the seventh grade, after six straight years spent wearing green knee socks and a plaid uniform, I switched from Catholic school to public school, where I felt even more out of place than before. It was 1998 and girls wore makeup, bellbottom jeans, and platform shoes. They chewed gum, spoke out, even cursed in class. The boys were just as much of a leap in the opposite direction of what I was used to. There were sporty kids and preppy kids and drug dealer kids (I had won a D.A.R.E. essay contest in the fifth grade, and up until this point, I thought drugs were something I would never encounter in real life). Everyone seemed to be part of a tightknit clique or a gang, and as far as I was concerned, they were all aliens from another planet. Needless to say, I felt culture-shocked and naive, ill-equipped to navigate this strange new land of pubescent people.

I remember shaking, literally shaking with social anxiety, before I knew what social anxiety even was. I trembled in the hallways and in all my classes each time a teacher made me read aloud or uttered the dreaded phrase, "Everybody find a partner." My stomach was perpetually twisting, tightening around its own knots.

THE PRESSURES OF PUBERTY

About halfway through my adolescence, I suddenly felt an enormous amount of pressure to find a boyfriend, to experience my first kiss, and to start experimenting with my body. Suddenly, *everyone* at school was dating, not just the first-to-bloom kids at the top of the social totem pole. But for me, there were obstacles. For starters, my hormones weren't making me hungry for boys. Second, I still didn't have an "in" with any particular group of people in my grade, nor was I willing to participate in contrived social activities like pep rallies and school dances. And third, possibly the biggest hurdle of all, was that I knew that in order to engage in any of these new experiences, I would have to become a *woman* in my parents' eyes.

The thought of growing up felt somehow taboo to me, as if in doing so, I'd be letting down two of the only people I'd ever truly cared for. I'm not entirely sure what led me to feel this way. It could've been because both of my parents were very involved in my life and seemed very attached to being parents, and so perhaps I was afraid I'd hurt them if I was no longer their little girl. My home life and the role I played in my family as a child was the only comfort I'd ever really known. My parents' love and approval was my greatest sense of security and self-esteem.

I grew up with one sibling, my twin sister, Kristy, and we had similar feelings of guilt attached to our impending developing selves. I recall, for example, hoping to God that Kristy would get her period for the first time before I did so that she could pioneer coping with the shame and embarrassment that would come with it. But sure enough, one day while playing volleyball in gym class, I felt a painful, burning sensation between my legs, and when I went to the bathroom, all I saw was red. Of course I panicked. I purchased a Kotex pad from the cold metal vending machine for feminine products (thank all the goodness in the world it wasn't empty, and that I found a quarter in my book bag). Moments later, I found myself on a payphone with my mom, voice trembling, completely mortified, confessing to her that I was having my "time of the month" for the first time. My mom's voice on the other end of the line was motherly and joyful. "We'll have to celebrate when you get home," she said. But I was afraid of what that celebration would entail. In fact, now that I was bleeding like a woman, I couldn't imagine how life would go on.

This mortification around my femininity surfaced in many other ways as well. For one, I always felt awkward changing in front of other girls in the gym locker room. Long before it ever occurred to me I might be attracted to women, I felt "naughty" for being able to see other females undressing in my peripheral vision. My body was a different body—not like theirs. My discomfort with my own parts was furthered by the fact that I didn't shave my legs or armpits until high school, so I dreaded wearing shorts that would expose my hairy limbs.

In the lunchroom, boys would approach me from time to time, and it was always the same story: "Hi, my friend thinks you're cute. He's sitting over there. He wants to know if you'd like to go out sometime." I always said no without looking, unable to imagine uttering the phrase to my parents, "I'm going out with a boy." I was equally incapable of imagining myself batting my eyelashes and flirting playfully with a seventh-grade boy. I just wasn't ready.

Things got confusing when I became friends with a girl named Jessica. Jessica was slightly more popular than I was. In my mind, she was my ticket into a higher popularity bracket, and so making sure she liked me was important. The problem was that every time Jessica was around me, I'd become filled with a paralyzing anxiety. When the second period bell rang, I'd begin trembling, knowing I was going to see her in my third period typing class. Eventually, I started going over to Jessica's house and she would occasionally come over to mine. We did basic things together—played checkers, played video games, and ate dinner with either her parents or mine.

I don't recall there being anything profound about our friendship, nor did we ever become particularly close. But it's funny the way people sometimes enter our lives just to teach us things about ourselves. It's funny the way a moment can shift you. One day I went over to Jessica's house just as she and her mom were getting home from the grocery store. I went to the trunk of the car to help carry some of the groceries, but Jessica smiled and refused to allow me to help. Instead, she grabbed every plastic bag, her arms overloaded, and all I could think was, "That's hot." I don't know why, or where the thought came from. But it turned me on somewhere in my body, the fact that she took it upon herself to spare me from this one silly chore. Days later, I woke up from a dream where Jessica was on top of me, making out with me. And all I thought was, "That's interesting."

MY PARENTS' INFLUENCE

Here's something I've come to accept: we can't deny the ways in which we are shaped by our upbringings—regardless of the intentions of our caretakers. Our parents play an undeniably significant role in influencing our personalities, our temperaments, and the ways we come to view the world, especially when we are young. Also, we are shaped by more than our experiences—we're shaped by the *meaning* we assign to those experiences. That said, my parents are two of the most loving people on this earth and I'm grateful beyond words for them both. But I'd be leaving out an important part of my story if I didn't include their effect on me as a teenager.

My mom was the primary caretaker for my sister and I throughout our developing years, while my dad worked very long hours as a salesman. She carried much of the burden of caring for two twin girls, often on her own, and dedicated much of her life to our wellbeing. Perhaps because of this, she was very overprotective of my sister and I growing up—nothing I did made it past her, and in her mind, imminent danger was always just ahead. As kids, my sister and I weren't allowed to go over to our friends' houses for sleepovers unless my mom met and approved of each friend's parents—while this may have been appropriate for a period of time, it went on until we were well into our teens. She warned us time and again not to go to public bathrooms alone, not to talk to strangers, and to stay away from large, windowless vans. She opted to be a chaperone on most school trips; otherwise, we just wouldn't go. There were times my sister and I even caught my mom listening in on phone calls with our friends.

While I understand now that my mom's overly suspicious nature was rooted in her intention to keep me healthy and safe, as a young teenager with very little life experience, I had not yet reached the vantage point from which I could appreciate my mom's intense involvement in my life for what it was. I knew only that I was anxious, confused, and curious about so many things still beyond my conception. I came to believe that freedom was dangerous. Freedom came with a price tag, and so it was difficult for me to develop an early sense of who I was. Nonetheless, the last thing I wanted to do was disappoint my mom, and so I made it my responsibility to earn her approval at any cost, even when it meant sacrificing my own need for more independence.

As for my dad, his larger-than-life personality has always been endearing, but it felt a bit intrusive to me as a sensitive adolescent as I struggled to connect with the quiet depths that would later define me. My dad has the kind of carelessly extroverted presence that spills all over the place, fills up rooms, and dominates the spaces he enters. As a child, my dad was my hero—the guy who took me to experience new things and made everything more fun and exciting. He made snowmen with me in the snow, played volleyball with me in the pool, and gave me piggyback rides on the living room carpet. But when the disease of becoming a woman set in, I had the sense that my dad didn't know how to involve himself in my life in ways that would support my evolving emotional needs at the time.

BRANCHING OUT AS AN INDIVIDUAL

Although my sister and I had been around one another constantly for all our childhood years, by the time we reached high school, we each began to branch out more as individuals. No longer did we share the exact same friends, musical tastes, or clothing styles (pretty much the only things that matter when you're a teenager). But this is not to say we "grew apart," necessarily. Instead, the distance felt more like an unspoken agreement between our souls. The need to grow as separate beings and the desire to explore our budding selves had become too intense at this point to ignore. And although we were not yet mature enough to confide everything in one another throughout the rocky phases of self-discovery, in time, our separate journeys actually brought us closer.

When it came to socializing, Kristy and I were a little bit different. Kristy attempted to break away from a contained upbringing by having adventures with new people who enabled her to feel a new sense of freedom and possibility. I, on the other hand, went out and socialized in more conservative ways, cautiously collecting new experiences and reflecting on them. Kristy had different ways of dealing with her growing pains, too. She, a degree more rebellious than I, would wage wars with my parents, especially my mom, in the name of her independence. I remember angst-filled yelling matches during which my sister would argue for her God-given right to stay out past ten o' clock, while my mother retorted back at her that she could live on her own if she wanted to make her own rules. I was different in that I avoided confrontation at all costs. Instead, I internalized a lot of my feelings and let fear control most of my decisions until eventually I did what all teenagers do. I started telling white lies to protect my parents from who I needed to become.

Another layer of oppression many people experience as adolescents has to do with society. My sister, who is a psychotherapist now, agrees that while adolescents are typically stereotyped as bratty or narcissistic in their quest to discover who they are, the need to formulate an identity at this age is so critical. And yet, it's precisely at this age that we are first plagued with many responsibilities of adulthood. It's no wonder so many teenagers are moved to rebel and express themselves through radical means; they're not given the room to explore themselves as they go through one of the biggest transitions of their lives. Instead, society places all this weight on their shoulders.

Another important element to take into consideration here is that not every teenager's temperament is the same. My sister and I have always been exceptionally deep, observant, highly sensitive people. So our need to reflect and take our time with developing was perhaps even greater than for the average person. Not having this time caused me a great deal of overwhelm and anxiety.

HALLELUJAH, I'M A LESBIAN

I didn't date anyone until the eleventh grade. My first boyfriend, Joe, had sweaty hands and a frog-like face. He wore emo glasses, played guitar, and listened to Green Day. As horrible as it is to say, my agreeing to date Joe was more of an "all right, let's get this boyfriend thing over with" thing than anything based on any sort of attraction. I remember my first kiss. Joe and I were at the movies, and we'd planned to plant our mouths on one another's for the first time as soon as the lights went dark in the theater. He'd just finished eating a Butterfinger, and I could smell the candy on his breath before I tasted it. It was an unremarkable kiss, devoid of sparks, triggering zero emotions (at least on my end). But the possibility that I might be a lesbian still had yet to cross my mind. I had so little experience socially and romantically that I chalked up the lack of fireworks to the fact that I was a novice, that I hadn't yet discovered "my type," or that I wasn't popular enough to attract someone I could actually be attracted to.

Shortly after Joe came Mike and Jon and Chris and Matt. To me, they were all the same. I went through the motions of what I thought it meant to flirt, though I was only mimicking what I saw other

girls doing and it came with extreme discomfort.
I don't know how else to describe the role I felt
forced into each time I sat in the passenger seat of
a guy's car, except to say that I felt in every sense
a passenger. Next to men, I have always felt as if I
should be expected to concede...to their agendas, to
their ideas, and to their physical desires. They were
never in tune with me emotionally; instead, they had
a predetermined sense of how I should fit myself into
their lives. Even when certain guys worshipped me
for my intelligence and qualities I appreciate being
noticed for, it still felt as if I was this "thing" to them,
an accessory they could show off and from which they
could derive satisfaction.

My realizing-I-was-gay story is funny, in that it
was literally a realization I came to overnight. I was
dating Matt at this point, a fairly decent looking boy
I had met in acting class. Sometimes on school nights
Matt would pick me up in his van to go to the local
diner for "hot chocolate." What this really meant is
that I'd watch him stuff his face with a disgusting
cheeseburger, and then he'd ask me for a blowjob in
the parking lot.

Eventually came the day our acting class took
a field trip to see *Wicked* on Broadway, and Matt

introduced me to his friend Cat. Within seconds of meeting Cat, I felt as if I had known her for years. There was something familiar and endearing about her—perhaps I was sensing echoes of my future self, already aware she would shape my life in a way that would forever shift me. But never before had I felt so instantly compatible with another person. Cat was bubbly and affectionate; she laughed at the things I said and made me feel comfortable in my skin.

One night shortly after we met, Cat and I were chatting on AOL instant messenger when the possibility occurred to me that I might be attracted to women. Matt was constantly flirting with other girls. The status of having a boyfriend was the only part of being with Matt that actually appealed to me. Other than that, he didn't make my heart beat any faster. Something just wasn't right. Struck with the sudden urge to confide in someone, I told Cat how I'd been feeling. To my surprise, Cat replied, "I've been wondering the same thing about myself." And with that, we agreed to "test" ourselves out on one another, despite both having boyfriends. The very next night, Cat came over, and after a few shots of vodka borrowed from my parents' liquor cabinet, she leaned in to me and said, "I told you I wouldn't be afraid."

Then we kissed, and electricity ran through every part of my body. Overcome with a combination of lust and shame, I felt desire for the first time. I wanted more.

For a moment, I sought refuge in my new discovery. I asked myself, *Is this why I've felt different all my life? Because I'm a lesbian? Is this why I've never felt like other girls?* Suddenly, everything made sense. I could read the writing on the wall.

Now that I'd resolved this tremendous part of my identity, I finally felt motivated to take the risks required to get to know myself more intimately. This is when I began to tell more substantial lies to my parents, like the time I said I was staying at a friend's house for the day so I could take an Amtrak to Philadelphia to visit Alex, a girl I had met online, and experiment with her sexually; or the several times I snuck out my bedroom window, or smuggled a girl in through it. It was all pretty harmless, honestly. But it was harmful in the way that each time I told a lie, I reinforced something terrible in my own mind: that I had to keep secrets in order to get what I wanted.

MY SISTER'S ENCOUNTER WITH SELF-HARM

Unbeknownst to me, around the time I discovered I liked girls, my sister had discovered the same thing about herself. In fact, she'd been discreetly fooling around with a girl for a couple of months (I'll call the girl "Hanna") and was in the midst of having her heart broken for the very first time. As I found out from my sister later, Hanna was moody, mentally unstable, and perhaps sexually confused. She took Kristy on a lust-filled roller coaster ride only to eventually go back to her boyfriend, leaving Kristy in the dust. The fling ended dramatically and abruptly with Hanna being hospitalized for cutting herself.

The day I found out what Kristy had gone through was the day my mom noticed scabbed streaks of red emerging from Kristy's long-sleeved shirt and demanded that she roll back her sleeves to expose her forearms. Kristy refused as adamantly as I'd ever heard her refuse anything, but my mom persisted until she finally forced Kristy to reveal her arms. The gasp that came from my mom next was the gasp that changed everything. My sister had cut herself deeply with a box cutter—so deeply, in fact, that she has scars to this day.

Recently, I asked my sister's permission to include this part of the story in this book and also asked her if she could tell me more. She sent me the following in a text:

"I did it because I was in pain and it didn't seem like anyone really knew. I was a depressed, closeted homo in love with a very disturbed yet very alluring girl. I did it because I felt trapped. Seeking support around this would have meant 'coming out' and I just wasn't ready for all that yet. I wasn't even sure yet myself what I was. At the time I was aware that in a sick way I wanted Hanna to find out what I'd done to myself. I wanted her to know how much I cared about her and how hurt I was about her hurting herself. I wanted her to see her own reflection in me. I wanted her to see that perhaps we were more alike than she knew. In a weird way, cutting myself brought me to terms with the level of pain and numbness I was experiencing. The fact that I could harm myself to such an extent and barely feel it was evidence of my suffering, and so was the blood. It was proof of my existence, and so are the scars."

After my sister's encounter with self-harm, there was a significant shift in my family's dynamics. My mother and father, concerned as any parents would be, took every measure they could to prevent Kristy from hurting herself again, from an initial trip to the emergency room to getting Kristy enrolled into psychotherapy. Patronizing doctors and concerned family members asked my sister, "Why would you do this to your precious skin?" Eventually, my mom sought treatment of her own and began seeing a therapist for a time, who I think pushed her to let Kristy and I have more trust and independence. This ultimately led to my mom pulling back and giving Kristy and I more room to grow as individuals.

My sister and I came out as gay a couple of years later, and my parents actually took the news lovingly and well. But still we had this in common: our first notions of romantic love were that it involved things we had to conceal. Euphoria and joy were feelings to be ashamed of, feelings we had to steal.

Chapter 2
MY QUARTER-LIFE CRISIS

-

In this section, I'll tell you about the events that immediately preceded what I refer to as "my big fat discreet breakdown," which occurred less than six months into my first year away at college. It was some combination of feeling for the first time like I was free, combined with the pressures of new expectations—social expectations, adult responsibilities, etc.—which I did not yet know how to navigate. All the while I was experiencing this sense of overwhelm, I was also yearning, reaching, searching for something I could not quite put my finger on. And so I challenged everything—my sexuality, my metaphysical body, and my desires—essentially, my entire identity.

OVERWHELMED BY THE LIMITLESS WORLD

The year I turned eighteen, I sought many things—freedom from my social anxiety, control over my feelings and desires, and relief from the pressure to *become* someone in a world that made little sense to me. In what felt like a very short span of time, I was expected to choose a four-year college, commit to a career path, assume a personality, and assert myself in ways I just wasn't prepared for. For years, I had mastered the art of being invisible—and now I was expected to be someone? It was too much to ask, it was too much, too soon, and I wanted nothing more than to retreat into a private corner and hide.

The way I see it, when you're a child, the world is big and that's okay because it's far away. When you're all grown up, the world is smaller and more manageable because you've carved your shape into it, so you need only to live in that shape. But when you're stuck in that awkward space between childhood and adulthood, it's like being a fly in a windstorm, trying to navigate a limitless sky while gusts of wind blow at you from every direction. I was still trying to get my shit together, far too curious to commit to anything, let alone an identity. I was simply *hungry* for so many things I could not yet define.

BEGINNING TO PLAY WITH MY FOOD

It was around this time that I started to become really curious about my body. Although I wasn't overweight to begin with (maybe five pounds at most), I saw dieting as an opportunity to escape myself, to distract myself, and to gain some handle of control over the fast-approaching demands of adulthood. I just wanted to feel like I was moving toward something measurable and meaningful without having to actually deal with real life. It was innocent at first. I started replacing cookies and chips with fruit, Melba toast, and other things that tasted like cardboard, which seemed like a commendable thing to do. I bought a couple of diet books from a local thrift store, both from the 1980s, and did my best to consume zero percent fat whenever possible.

The summer I graduated high school, I enrolled in a summer film program at NYU and lived in a dorm room by myself for a month and a half in the West Village of New York City. I had never taken a subway before, I had no idea how to get around, and I felt this enormous sense of possibility combined with loneliness and paralysis. More than anything, I remember not knowing how to feed myself. *Nobody's watching*, I kept thinking to myself. *Nobody's watching me at all.* That meant I could do, say, or consume whatever I wanted, and there would be no real repercussions aside from those I decided to impose upon myself. Iced coffee for breakfast? Pop tarts for lunch? Sure, if I wanted to. This feeling of being totally on my own was something I had never experienced before in my life, and I had no clue how to fill the void.

It's a cliché I'm trying to avoid, to color eating disorders as diseases born out of superficiality that erupt in the minds of girls with low self-esteem who read too many issues of *CosmoGirl* magazine, but I do recall being struck by a particular billboard one evening on my walk back from shooting reels around the city. It was a billboard image of the actress Shannyn Sossamon, who was scrawny and edgy with a protruding collarbone and black eye make up that gave her "raccoon eyes," and I remember thinking, *That. I want to be that.* The distinction I need to articulate is that for me, it was not the idea of being *scrawny* that I romanticized necessarily, but rather the idea of being *broken*. Scrawny was just part of what it meant to be broken. Deciding to skip dinner, I wondered how long I might be able to go without eating anything at all. And with that, the void lessened. With that, the void became me.

COLLEGE, THE EXISTENTIAL QUEST

In September of 2005, I went away to Purchase College in Westchester, New York, a school known for being artsy, liberal, and open-minded, and felt I had found my tribe at last. Hipsters, freaks, and queers scattered around campus in their band T-shirts and skinny jeans, smoking cigarettes like they were famous. They carried cameras and portfolios, and at least half of them had some combination of brightly colored hair, tattoos, and facial piercings. I remember reading in one online review about Purchase that it was the "college for dodgeball targets." But if that was the case, then dodgeball targets were my favorite kind of people. Finally, I was surrounded by artists, writers, actors, and dancers—people with substance and eccentricities I could relate to and admire. And for the first time in my life, people my age actually took an interest in my thoughts and ideas. A good handful even found me intriguing. Even my professors were progressive, unique individuals who embraced the school's motto, "Think wide open."

One particularly definitive memory I have of Purchase happened my first week as a freshman. It was the hottest September I had ever encountered, and I remember tossing, turning, and sweating on the

springy top bunk mattress of my dorm room, relieved
only by the most compact of compact fans. Then,
one night, after days of the humidity building and
building so that the campus felt like it was swelling like
a mother ready to give birth, the sky cracked open and
it began pouring rain like it had never rained before.
The sense of new beginnings was in the air, prompting
every freshman to leap up and run outside, barefoot,
naked—anything went. They laughed and danced and
did cartwheels in the grass as if they had just arrived on
this planet, as if they had never experienced rain before
in their lives. I stood watching, my chest pounding
a kind of euphoric melody, and debated what to do
with my body. I felt, for a split second, like I could
jump around, dance, and do cartwheels if I wanted to.
I could finally let *go*. But the possibility only flickered
in me like a trying, reluctant flame. And the most I
could bring myself to do was stand there, completely
paralyzed, terrified of looking like a fool.

For the first couple of months of my first semester,
I continued to feel enamored by the new people
and ideas that surrounded me. I was so enamored in
fact that I decided to break up with my first serious
girlfriend, who was still living back home on Long
Island. I was in love with Meghan right up until the

day I ended our relationship (in fact, far, far beyond that day). Yet, there was an appetite in my soul that was somehow bigger than that love. I had been committed to Meghan for nearly two years. She represented all the comforts of home and embodied many of the traits I wanted in a partner, but in my heart, I knew I had to explore myself and this exciting new chapter of my life without limitation. I was searching for something that was even deeper than the intimacy I could share with a romantic partner.

It was around this time that I began a mad love affair with philosophy, particularly existentialism. Existentialism, as defined by the Merriam-Webster dictionary, is a branch of philosophy which is characterized by the analysis of individual existence in an unfathomable universe and the plight of the individual, who must assume ultimate responsibility for acts of free will without any certain knowledge of what is right or wrong or good or bad. I got carried away with questions that would unravel my entire reality: Do I have free will or is everything predetermined? What do I actually believe in, and in what ways are all of my beliefs the result of conditioning? Is there such a thing as an absolute truth, or is my entire reality a projection of my biased perceptions? When am I my authentic self and when am I performing? What is *real*?

I formed friendships with people who asked the same questions, and our favorite thing to do was to sit somewhere on the grass under the stars, smoking cigarettes and breaking down the entirety of our existence until there was nothing left to ponder.

One night in the campus courtyard, my friend Jen pointed at the sky and said, "Look at the moon."

"Yes, wow, it's so big and yellow," I replied.

"No, it isn't big or yellow," Jen said. "It just *is*."

"What do you mean, 'it just *is*?'"

"It just *is*," Jen replied. "You'll get it someday."

As I later understood, what Jen was trying to communicate to me that night is that there's a truth in things we can feel when we're able to look at things, especially things in nature, without judgment. Nothing can be truly understood. And yet, there's a special kind of peace that comes with surrendering to the mystery and wonder of creation. There's freedom in the kind of mindful awareness that doesn't try to own or control or identify various aspects of existence. To truly experience the moon, or anything for that matter, we must simply allow things to be what they are.

I'm afraid, however, that before I was able to truly grasp this concept, I misinterpreted it. I decided that if the moon wasn't big or yellow, then I wasn't anything either. I was personality-less, identity-less, sexuality-less. I was just a body that could not be labeled or defined. I tried on different personas for a time, seeing how people would respond. One day I could be quiet, mysterious, and aloof, and the next I could be talkative. I felt unguided by any sense of intuition– I was just a game piece, and life was just a game.

SECOND GUESSING GAY

Never once in my life have I felt a raw, animalistic attraction toward a male. That shy, googly-eyed thing that happens to people when they're crushing— I've had it for girls, but never for the other side. Nonetheless, there came a point for me where I worried about the *what ifs. What if* I hadn't given guys a fair shot when I dated them before? *What if* I'd never experienced a boy I had things in common with or found aesthetically attractive? *What* if there was something about the boys in my high school, the boys of Long Island, that didn't turn me on, but I could feel feelings for guys with more substance from more interesting places? I never doubted my interest in girls, but since I was newly single and challenging my mind to be wide open, as it were, I figured why not put my sexuality back on the table.

Shortly thereafter I was approached in the campus library by a suave Visual Arts major named Craig. Craig was by far the most attractive member of the male species that had ever expressed interest in me; he was tall with a medium build, sandy hair, and proportionate facial features. He was focusing on metal sculpture at the time, which meant he welded metal with a blowtorch into sculptures as tall as he was (pretty badass, I thought). Craig hit the mark with the way he introduced himself to me, too, with a well-executed blend of humor and swag. *Yes, he will do*, I thought. *I will try him on for size.*

I went to Craig's dorm room a few times after that, and we made out to the soundtrack of Elliott Smith. We went out to dinner, seemingly had conversational chemistry, and talked about everything under the sun. Craig was intelligent, deep, and interesting—all the things I thought I "should" find attractive. And yet, each time he kissed me, I felt nothing but the stubble on his face. When he pushed himself against me, both of us fully clothed, it felt more forced than intimate. I felt no urge to pull his shirt over his head—no desire to expose his hairy man body.

Within weeks of Craig, my friend Tristan, a philosophy major, confessed that he had feelings for me despite my telling him from the time we met that I was a lesbian. Tristan and I had something sweet— the weather had turned cold by then, and so we'd spend many late nights together sitting on the dryers in the basement of my building, engaging in heated philosophical conversations until three in the morning. I could always tell Tristan was charmed by my ability to debate with him and keep up with the complicated theories he liked to throw at me. But I never expected he'd spill his heart to me the way he did. On this particular evening, Tristan and I had decided to hike up a small hill that was tucked alongside the campus. He waited until we'd made it to the top, then when we were finally sitting down admiring the view, still panting from the climb, he told me he loved me, with genuine tears behind his eyes.

My heart stuttered. Tristan was neither a bad-looking nor exceptionally good-looking guy. He was tall and lanky with black hair and an Adrian Brody nose. I didn't feel attracted to him, just as I didn't feel attracted to Craig, but felt more of an obligation to protect Tristan's feelings and let him down gently, given the weight of his confession. Eventually, I had to say the only true words that could find their way to my lips: "Tristan, I like you as a person and I value our friendship. But I'm gay. I've always been gay. I've told you this from the beginning."

But Tristan had a hard time understanding how he could feel something so strongly himself that wasn't reciprocated at all.

"Come with me," he said, as he took my hand. "I want to show you something."

And so I followed Tristan down the hill, into the darkness, and into an unlocked classroom in the middle of campus.

"Have a seat," Tristan said. "Any seat you like." And with that he proceeded to march to the front of the classroom, chalk in hand, ready to mimic a professor. Tristan had a mission and only one mission: to turn my "sexuality" into a philosophic debate. He wanted to challenge all the ways in which I'd been socially conditioned to believe I could only be attracted to women. He wanted to know what it was about his body—a body made only of meaningless matter—that prevented us from exploring one another on romantic terms. "Sexuality is only a construct of the mind," he said.

"Then why don't you go date men?" I replied. I offered counterarguments to all of Tristan's arguments, all the while laughing at how ridiculous he was being. But underneath the laughter, I wasn't laughing. I was enraged, mainly at myself for entertaining this person before me who was trying to strip me of my sexuality as if it were a mask I chose to wear out of stubbornness.

My intuition, which I had abandoned for too long, climbed up from my gut then, flushing my face with red, pulling the corners of my forced smile downward. It was the fuel I needed to walk away from Tristan, to walk away from Craig, to walk away from the notion that I should use logic to try and convince myself I "should" be with a man, or that I "should" be anything I didn't want to be, for that matter. Logic did not speak the language of my bones.

Imagine a straight man having to force himself to be with another man, or a straight woman having to force herself to be with another woman– it would feel uncomfortable for them and foreign. It'd probably even make them feel violated. But a good majority of queer people feel pressure from society to challenge their intuitive instincts in this way—to experiment with the opposite sex to "make sure" they aren't "normal" before accepting themselves as different. I've since used this analogy to describe it: imagine you were born into the world as it is, and you were able to fly. Now, ninety-five percent of the people around you walk on the ground. There is just a small percentage of people like you who can fly, too, but the people on the ground are always trying to make them feel bad about it. The people on the ground say, "The bible says flying is a sin. Keep flying and you'll fly your way straight into hell." But flying is the most exhilarating part of your life—the only thing that makes you feel truly you. Would you fly without ever once doubting yourself? Or would you, at least at first, buy into the idea that something might be wrong with you? Would you hide your wings and walk on the ground?

It's quite toxic, especially for a developing person, to be conditioned to believe they need to conform to the majority in order to be worthy of love and acceptance. Yes, I wished, for the sake of my own curiosity and for the sake of understanding the world around me, that I could understand for just once in my life what it might feel like to desire a guy. But how unreasonably generous of me to sacrifice my body and my truth in order to satisfy somebody else's idea of what is moral and normal and right.

I adore women. To this day, I'm not sure how I identify myself, but one thing I know for certain is that when I make love to a woman, I am faceless and genderless—lost in the exhilaration of her soft curves, the balanced way that power shifts between us, and the unspoken understanding between two female minds. Nothing in fact feels more spiritual to me than being with another woman in this way. In making love to a woman, I feel the presence of God.

MY BIG FAT DISCREET BREAKDOWN

All in all, philosophy, along with the way I challenged everything I knew to be true, including the ground beneath my feet, was too much for a person whose sense of self was already so dangerously fragile. To this day I have a love for debating with others over life's biggest questions, but at my young age then, I just wasn't ready. I had enough trouble as it was deciding what kind of cereal to eat in the morning, let alone addressing the existential crises of humankind.

By the end of my first semester at Purchase, my mind had been filled with the weightlessness of so many ideas that it started to ascend from my shoulders like a helium balloon, completely disconnecting from my body. I didn't know what to say or how to act. I spent time with whoever wanted to spend time with me, never exercising my own agency by choosing to surround myself with people who actually made me feel happy. Not surprisingly, I wasn't able to stand up for myself, since I didn't know how to stand for anything at all, and so I was only floating. What I was dealing with was a kind of intellectual boundlessness combined with emotional paralysis. I had allowed myself to develop too rapidly on a cerebral level without maturing my other layers. And so I had no ability to be vulnerable or expressive. All I was able to share with others were my questions and ideas, which ultimately led nowhere at all.

Eventually, I had to face the grim reality that I had very few people in my life I could call true friends—just a storm of acquaintances, most of whom were intrigued by me only for the mysterious persona I projected. Who was I? I still didn't know. I felt grounded in nothing, unhinged from a world in which everyone else seemed to participate so effortlessly. This thing in me that had always felt different somehow still felt different, even amongst like-minded people. And at the end of every day, I was alone.

With all of that, I began to feel I'd made a huge mistake in breaking up with Meghan, and I wanted to punish myself for my greed, for not realizing how special my relationship had been, and for desiring new experiences. Had I been too impulsive? Had I made a huge mistake? Simultaneously I felt the gravity of how much I missed my family, which is something I hadn't really been acknowledging. I missed the feeling of their love and attention being there every day. Now everything that mattered to me, everything safe and familiar, was light-years away. As these feelings flooded over me like a violent tsunami, Purchase, this magical place full of wonder and possibility, lost all of its color. November came. The leaves began to fall, monochrome against the gray earth. And as the air grew thick and cold, so did my will to move forward.

Suspecting I was more than superficially depressed, by the middle of December the day came when I found the nerve to walk myself down to the campus psychotherapy office wearing only a T-shirt (what is cold anyway, but a construct of the mind?). I met with a counselor who didn't seem to take me seriously when I confessed to her that I felt nothing. I felt completely numb. And I was beginning to struggle with eating. She appeared to me to be worn out by many years of work; I sensed that her heart was not in it. Her raisin skin puckered beneath too many layers of makeup, and her eyes were absent, surrounded by smudged black liner. When I told her the act of putting food in my mouth made me feel the weight of infinity upon my bones, she took a few notes on her yellow pad and responded without flinching that I looked a little too thin but that the feelings I was feeling seemed very normal.

I returned to my dorm room more hopeless than before, set on the fact that I needed to explore myself through some other means; I had to get to the bottom of what I was feeling, and I had to do it on my own. That evening, filled with apathy and delirium, I laced up my sneakers and went for a run in the pouring rain. I ran to relieve the riptides in my chest, the yearning for a thing I still couldn't put my finger on. Pacified by the meditation of one foot in front of the other, I ran until I couldn't feel my legs, until the world around me melted into puddles and stardust.

Chapter 3
MY SECRET BATTLE
WITH FOOD

-

In chapters 3 and 4, I'll take you through the dark days of my eating disorder from the moment it erupted fully. This includes the silly games I played with myself to help me starve my body more "successfully," my compulsive addiction to exercise, and my eventual struggle with bulimia. It all leads up to a climatic moment where things began to shift for the better—the first time I witnessed what it feels like to be present in my body and surrender to what is beyond my control.

A DAY IN THE LIFE OF AN EATING DISORDER

Beyond overstimulated, I left Purchase after that first semester in 2005 and retreated to my parents' house to hibernate in the spaces where I could be inconspicuous again—the privacy of my bedroom, my car, and wherever else I'd be preserved rather than observed by the eyes of others. Upon returning home, my curiosity about life, fate, and everything else intensified into something dangerous and self-defeating. I finally had a minute to breathe, but still, all I could think about was running. So, I literally continued to run—first a lap around my parents' block, then two, until I was able to do six laps every day without stopping. Finally, I had the privacy and space to indulge in a ritualistic lifestyle that would enable me to distract myself from my emotions, and what that manifested as for me was a full-fledged eating disorder.

I began to starve myself very strategically and deliberately and exercised as often as I possibly could. It was all I could think to do to diffuse my anxiety and push away the black cloud that was now looming over me. I hated myself for failing at socializing and for being incapable of relating to others. I hated myself for feeling paralyzed in the face of too many decisions about a future that felt uncertain. And now, I had too much time on my hands.

I enrolled in community college to complete my associate degree, but nothing I studied intrigued me more than my new obsession. I sat in class calculating the calories I had eaten so far that day as hunger pangs beat at my insides. I couldn't focus on anything except the void in the pit of my stomach and the strange sense of calm that came with that pain.

The ritual was the same each morning. I'd wake up, strip off my pajamas, and step onto the scale. Wherever the needle stopped would determine my level of self-esteem for the day, and gaining weight was not an option. Next, I'd lace up my running sneakers and sprint three or four miles on an empty stomach. I was addicted to the high—the lightheadedness that came first, then the pleasant, euphoric feeling of being as light as air, surrounded by a blur of trees and houses and sky. No longer was I limited by a body. I was one with the universe, one with creation, *free*.

When I went to the gym, it was always for an hour or more, and I'd work out as hard as I possibly could, even when I was tired or sick. No physical obstacle could compete with my emotional *need* to burn calories. I was ruthless toward myself, as if I had some sort of indomitable courage that enabled me to push my body to limits I never imagined possible. Comforted by the humdrum repetition of feet pounding against the treadmill, I'd close my eyes and zone out for sixty straight minutes, then bask in the glow of the red numbers flashing: *600 calories burned.*

Like a mad scientist, I calculated every calorie and every morsel of food before it entered my mouth. I spent hours at health food stores carefully probing ingredient lists, and purchased only products I considered "safe foods." Most days, I ate a carefully measured three-fourths cup of bran cereal for breakfast, a piece of fruit and coffee for lunch, and something light for dinner, such as salad, fat-free cottage cheese, or a cereal bar. I used coffee, cigarettes, and large glasses of water as vices to suppress my appetite. To get myself "energized" before the gym, I invested in every supplement on the market—caffeine pills, ginseng, and an assortment of powders and tinctures.

The whole of me was governed by a series of self-imposed rules and rituals, such as "no eating within three hours of bedtime," "no eating between planned 'meals,'" and "no carbs after six o'clock." In addition, I'd manifested a series of non-food-related OCD behaviors; for example, it took me two hours to leave the house, because I had developed rituals associated with getting ready. I'd have to check three times to make sure my flat iron was off, then three times to make sure the oven was off. I didn't trust myself to make it out the door without forgetting something terribly important, and there was no room for deviation or compromise—everything had to be the way I had decided it should be. If anything got in the way of my plan, I'd feel irreparably defeated and shut off from contact with the world.

The less I consumed, the less I was able to consume, and the more I exercised, the more determined I became to raise the bar even higher. It was a game to me to see how creatively and imaginatively I could trick my body into taking the abuse. But as I got sucked deeper and deeper into the vortex, my body was changing on a physiological level too. At five foot eight, I had dwindled down to a muscular 112 pounds. My period stopped, and with that, I lost my lust for many things. With fewer than a thousand calories a day to sustain me, my thinking became even more disorganized, and I had difficulty focusing. I became spacey and detached, awash with an even deeper apathy that shifted my reality into a sick maze I couldn't escape from.

I became so disconnected from my body, so removed from its natural cues of hunger and satiation, that I could no longer remember what eating normally even felt like. It was as if I was drowning in an ocean that had no surface. After manipulating the meaning of nourishment for so long, I could no longer tell which way was up and which way was down—what was feeding me and what was destroying me. There was a war inside my head that said I needed to hurt myself to survive.

Yes, I became completely preoccupied with my appearance, because that *is* part of the disease, but it didn't stem from a place of vanity. As I mentioned before, it's too much of a cliché to say every girl who gets an eating disorder is brainwashed by western standards of beauty. I was never one of those girls who thumbed through the pages of girly magazines, mouth hanging open in awe, wishing I could be gaunt like the models so that I could be beautiful. Instead, I was obsessed with my reflection in the mirror because I no longer identified with my body. My body felt foreign to me, like this picture projected before my eyes that I could decide to believe in or not.

I remember standing in the kitchen one day when my sister looked at me with a blend of horror and disgust. She told me she could see every vertebra of my backbone through my t-shirt. At first, the comment inflated me with a sense of achievement and pride. Then I wondered, *am I sick?* I needed to be more than thin to feel a sense of integrity with myself; I needed to be *emaciated*. Each time thereafter, when someone told me I looked too skinny, I'd play it off just as nonchalantly, then smile hugely inside my fragile heart. But beyond these rare moments of gratification, I was chronically unfulfilled, still aching to express the stubborn force within me.

Since I was living at home again, I did the best I could to maintain my ritualistic eating and exercise habits without giving my parents reason to become suspicious. To avoid evening meals, I had to make up excuses such as, "I ate already" or, "I'm going out for food later with friends." Of course this sent me into a perpetual guilt cycle. In an effort to control every variable of every situation, I had to push everyone and everything I loved away from me. Every ounce of my energy was directed toward maintaining my rituals and keeping the world from intruding. It was literally and emotionally exhausting. Social spontaneity became an impossibility. Joy was not something I even had a sense of anymore. I was just a racehorse running straight forward with blinders on, unable to see anything but the finish line.

One night, my parents asked me to join them for dinner at Ruby Tuesday and I was terrified. I had spent the entire morning and afternoon carefully controlling the amount of fat and calories I allowed to enter my body. I had gone to the gym and had run for forty-five minutes on the treadmill, then did half an hour of leg presses and squats, and I wasn't about to throw all of that hard work down the drain for a single meal from a chain restaurant. But I thought, *I can do it this time. Just this time.* So I wouldn't have to lie again.

As soon as we were seated in the booth, my eyes began diligently scanning the menu from front to back. The conversation at the table became muffled by my deep concentration as I dedicated every bit of my attention to the objective of finding a low-calorie entree. After a five-minute journey through lists of heavy meats, creamy pasta dishes, and baskets of burgers and fries, I thought I had found my salvation.

"I'll have the shrimp appetizer," I told the waiter, "as my meal."

I sat back in my seat, feeling noble in my decision, and expected a modest plate of clean protein that I could take a few bites of and then abandon. But to my dismay, when the portion arrived, six battered shrimps stared up at me, deep-fried and sizzling in breadcrumbs and oil. My lungs fluttered against my ribs and tried to fly out of my chest. I couldn't breathe. I wanted to cry, not only because there was no way in hell I was eating something fried, but because I didn't want to make a scene in front of my parents by confronting the waiter and sending back my plate.

I placed a shrimp into my mouth and felt my thighs expanding as the grease coated my tongue and the salt hit the back of my throat. I was no longer pure. I was no longer in control. My lips quivered, and a temper tantrum broke out in my gut as I forced myself to keep chewing. It required every reserve of my energy to conceal the irrational amount of frustration that overcame me. Everything I'd done at the gym that day was for nothing, for fucking nothing. Now I'd have to work out for two hours the next day to make up for this. I broke out of my trance for long enough to hear my dad trailing on about his new landscaper and found myself momentarily fascinated by the fact that three people can coexist together at the same table, engulfed by such different realities.

MY FIRST TIME IN THERAPY

Although my parents were probably unaware of how severe my condition actually was, they eventually expressed their concern about my weight and urged me to eat more.

"You could put on about ten or fifteen pounds," my dad would say.

"Are you sure you're eating enough?" my mom would ask in a concerned tone. Eventually, my mom offered to pay for me to go to weekly therapy sessions.

I spent each Tuesday after that cautiously composed on a scratchy gray sofa, opening up about the weight in my mind before a licensed social worker named Katherine. By this point, I really wanted to get better. I also wanted to let someone in on the very secretive life I was living, so psychotherapy was not something I was opposed to. Katherine diagnosed me with an eating disorder during our first session, which pleased me. From there, she asked me questions about my family and my romantic life. She'd ask me what I had eaten for breakfast and what I planned to eat for lunch. But none of that is what transformed me.

MISINTERPRETING EASTERN PHILOSOPHY

It wasn't until Katherine and I started having conversations about Eastern philosophy that things started to get interesting. A recurrent theme throughout my eating disorder, I realized, was the part that felt undeniably…spiritual. I was fascinated by Buddhism (or at least the way I interpreted Buddhism) as this idea that I could overcome my cravings and attachments and therein free myself from human suffering. During all the time I had spent bearing hunger pangs and grinding away at the gym, I was convinced that if I could just discipline my body for long enough, eventually I'd no longer be limited by a body. That doesn't mean I was hoping to die or anything like that. I wasn't. I was just enlivened by a sense of possibility that had no place in reality—this idea that I might transcend the weight of the world if only I kept on pushing. Unfortunately for me, I took it too far. I'd managed to convince myself that even my own flesh was superfluous. I became so intrigued by the idea of "emptying myself out" that I was wasting away.

So the harder I fought, the more I eventually suffered. I was so caught up in trying to control my pain that I had neglected to realize the extent to which it was controlling me. Sure, there were moments in which I felt invincible, moments that had me feeling as if I was riding on a purer plane of existence where I was one with the transience of life, death, and everything in between. But those moments were always fleeting. It was always just a matter of time before I'd return to my broken, mortal self. Then, like any junkie, I'd be crawling in my veins until I got my next fix.

According to the Four Noble Truths of Buddhism:

1. Life is suffering. The very nature of human existence is inherently painful. Because of the cyclical nature of death and rebirth, death does not bring an end to suffering.

2. Suffering has a cause: craving and attachment. Suffering is the result of our selfish craving and clinging. This in turn reflects our ignorance of reality.

3. Craving and attachment can be overcome. When one completely transcends selfish craving, one enters the state of Nirvana, and suffering ceases.

4. The path toward the cessation of craving
and attachment is an Eightfold Path which
includes the right understanding, purpose,
speech, conduct, livelihood, effort, alertness,
and concentration.

According to Buddhist teachings, nothing is
permanent and no form endures forever. No single
perceived manifestation fully expresses the supreme
reality. For the Buddhist, developing the right kind
of self-discipline offers a pathway out of delusion and
toward true awareness. Holding on to what does not
actually exist will only lead to suffering.[2] I'm not going
to dive any deeper into the principles of Buddhism
here, but I will say I misinterpreted many of them
and used Eastern philosophy as an excuse to *dissociate*
from anything "indulgent" including my most
fundamental appetite.

So, there was the day Katherine said to me,
"Look." She folded her hands in thought and stared
off pensively for a moment before meeting my eyes
again with hers. "There are a lot of people in this
world who could benefit from Eastern wisdom—from
disempowering their egos, from considering their

---

2. Toropov, Brandon; Buckles, Luke. *The Complete Idiot's Guide to World
Religions*. Philadelphia: Alpha, 2004.

lives from other perspectives, and from humbling themselves in these ways. However, I don't think you're one of these people. In fact, I think you've got the opposite challenge here. You need to allow yourself to be more attached, to embody and embrace the full spectrum of your emotions from anger to sadness to disappointment. You need to put less responsibility on yourself to dissect everything into a million little pieces and try to trust your intuition. Just let yourself be."

While I didn't fully grasp Katherine's advice until later in life, she planted a very important little seed in me. It was the first time anyone had given me permission to trust my instincts. I'd been influenced my entire life by the "should" factor—the "shoulds" of the education system, the "shoulds" of the Catholic faith, the "shoulds" of being a good daughter, and the "shoulds" of society. My heart and mind were caged in my conception of everything I thought I should be. Rarely had I considered who I actually was, what I desired for myself, or what I needed to thrive in the world.

At the end of each of our sessions, Katherine gave me a pre-packaged gluten-free brownie she had purchased from the local health food store. It was her way of helping me to eat sometimes for the sake of enjoying food, and to live sometimes for the sake of enjoying life. Before long, my glove compartment was full of these brownies. I just wasn't yet ready to totally transform. But I was profoundly moved by the gesture.

THE TRANSIENCE OF APPLE PIE

One night, my mom knocked on my bedroom door and asked in a soft, cherubic voice, "Mariss, you got a minute?"

Many thoughts ran through my mind, as I feared my mom was about to confront me head-on about my eating disorder. Or maybe she wanted to ask me how therapy was going, or why my bedroom door was always locked, or—

"I have something for you." My mom's voice interrupted my mental chatter, and when I opened the door, she handed me a warm slice of apple pie with a scoop of vanilla ice cream on top. I thanked her with wide eyes and a knotted stomach. I knew the pie was a symbol of my mom's love for me and her desire for me to be nourished and happy. I knew she missed me, and that she wanted to check up on me. And I knew more than anything there was no way in hell I could eat it.

I closed the door and sat staring at the pie for a good while until tears welled up in my eyes and rolled down my cheeks. I tried to muster up the courage to take a single forkful for my mother's sake, but couldn't. I felt crushed at the thought of wasting something she had put her precious energy into. As steam ascended from the innocent slice, the ice cream melted into a puddle of milk on the plate, and in that puddle, I saw my reflection through my mother's eyes. She just wanted me to be okay. She *always* has. I continued to cry as I contended with the pain of disappointing her, and after about five minutes, the steam stopped rising. *Why do things turn from hot to cold? Why is food there, then gone? Why does everything have to end?*

I looked in the mirror then and saw a shell of the person I used to be—the shape of my collarbone and my sunken eyes. In that brief moment of clarity, I saw what I was doing to myself. I saw the "normal" girl I used to be, now so far away.

Chapter 4
THE ROAD TO RECOVERY

-

"Our life is an apprenticeship to the truth that around every circle another can be drawn; that there is no end in nature, but every end is a beginning; that there is always another dawn risen on mid-noon, and under every deep a lower deep opens."
–Ralph Waldo Emerson

-

SOMEONE TO SHARE THE FIGHT WITH

It was any morning. I was at the gym, whittling away at what little fat there was left on my body while drowning my brain in an iPod playlist titled "Hardcore Fuck Shit." This morning in particular, I'd decided to attempt the most daunting piece of equipment at the gym, the vertical climber. The vertical climber is pretty literally what it sounds like—two pedals and two handles attached to a vertical track, and the repetitive motion of cranking your legs and arms up and down at a rapid pace can burn over eight hundred calories an hour.

"Hey," said a voice. I didn't hear it at first. Then I felt a tap on my shoulder. Caught off guard, I plucked my ear buds from my ears, the sound of Peaches', "Fuck the Pain Away," still blaring audibly through them. I turned around and there stood Steve, an older bodybuilder who resembled Poseidon with long silver hair pulled back into a ponytail and a neatly trimmed white beard. Steve was in his mid-fifties, was built like the Hulk, and seemed like the last person in the gym who would interrupt me.

"You're pretty fierce, kid," Steve said. "You know, you're the only other person in this gym I've ever seen attempt to use this thing. It isn't easy."

"Thanks," I replied, as a bead of sweat dripped from my brow. I shot him a polite stare, preserving my distance and anxious to resume my workout, but Steve wasn't finished.

"I've seen you work, kid," he said with an approving, fatherly smile. He proceeded to challenge me by suggesting I turn the resistance dial a quarter turn to the right every two minutes until a full twenty minutes was up.

"This," he said, "will give you a dynamite workout."

Normally, if this was any other asshole at the gym, I think I'd have brushed him off and continued at my merry pace. But there was something about Steve that made me want to take him up on the challenge. Though every muscle in my body was screaming after the first couple of quarter turns, I was determined not to let Steve down. As I cranked away, working harder than I had ever worked before, I glanced periodically over to the other side of the gym where Steve lifted monstrous barbells with all his might. After ten minutes, I was already cooked, but I thought, *Keep going, keep going*. Steve's determination became my motivation, and impressing him was suddenly the only thing I cared about. When the twenty minutes were up, I climbed off the machine, drenched in perspiration from head to toe. Then, as if I'd passed his test, Steve met me back on the floor and handed me a business card with his name and number on it: *Steve Shepherd, Personal Trainer.*

"Give me a buzz if you ever want to pump some iron together," he said.

"Sure," I replied, debating whether or not I meant it. I left the gym in a daze, pondering my interaction with this older man, this complete stranger. But I couldn't help but smile crookedly at the fact that someone had noticed me. Someone had finally noticed me.

From that day on, Steve and I became a team of blood, sweat, and tears. We met at the gym every morning promptly at 6:30 a.m.. I'd be "talked to" if I was even two or three minutes late, and I lived for the discipline.

"Too much partying last night, Riss?" Steve would ask. Then he'd laugh in his humble way and declare forty-five minutes of cardio to straighten me out. After that, we'd spend up to an hour pumping metal like I'd never pumped metal before. Steve taught me how to box and how to swing kettle bells. He taught me the proper way to do lateral pull-downs, stiff-leg deadlifts, shoulder presses, and every other exercise I had attempted before with plenty of conviction but incorrect form. He pushed me hard, never doubting my abilities, and I never doubted his commands.

"Thirteen, fourteen, one more, Riss. You can do it...and now I need five!"

Eventually, I became comfortable enough to yell back at Steve during his sets. He showed me how to "spot" him like a trainer and assist him in pushing out those final few repetitions until every vein in his neck popped and his face exploded with red intensity.

Beyond uplifting my spirit, Steve also encouraged me to eat more. Within the first week of working together, Steve requested that I record everything I eat in two days' time and bring him a list so he could see what I was consuming.

"Well, that's easy," I told him. I could have given him the list on the spot, since it wasn't difficult to recall a bowl of cereal for breakfast, raisins and a soy latte for lunch, and steamed broccoli for dinner. I ate the same "meals" every day. Steve looked at me without judgment, but with some concern.

"We gotta get you eating more protein, Riss," he said.

Before I met Steve, I maintained a diet that was completely fat-free. I had little concern for feeding my body the proper nutrients, and it hadn't occurred to me that there were foods you could eat to fuel a workout and foods you should eat to recover—most importantly, protein. Since my diet consisted mainly of simple carbohydrates and coffee, there was a lot of room for improvement. Steve influenced me as no one else at the time could have to "eat to grow," rather than starving myself to shrink. He helped me to believe in myself each time he said, "Open your eyes and look yourself in the eye in the mirror," as I squatted with a ninety-pound barbell on my shoulders. "This is *you* doing this work. This is *you*."

In just a few short months, Steve helped me transform my body from scrawny to muscular. I started to incorporate more beans, lean meats, and tofu into my diet. In no time at all, I was even able to drink vanilla Muscle Milk without any anxiety. Sure, it might have contained seven grams of fat, but I was okay with that. I had a new obsession now, and it was to be CUT.

As Steve and I became closer over time, our casual chitchats between sets grew into something more personal and bonding. If I was having an off day, I was able to talk with him about rough patches with girls I was dating, and he listened like an accepting parent. In exchange, Steve opened up to me about personal matters in his own life. One morning in particular, Steve asked if I minded sitting down with him for a moment. "Of course," I said and gulped hard, fearing what he might confess. Steve took a deep breath and looked somber—a far stretch from the Mr. Motivation he had always been. Then he told me, as if he'd been holding it inside of himself like a burning coal, that he was estranged from his teenaged daughter. With this confession, I watched Steve deflate completely. As a young girl who Steve had clearly taken a liking to, perhaps I should have been more put off by this news. *What could he have done to his daughter to cause her to estrange herself from him? Was he abusive? Did he hurt her?* But when I looked up again and saw Steve's face twist into something so broken and hollow, I felt only compassion. Maybe he had done nothing to deserve it at all, which might explain the passion and intensity he brought to his workouts. Or maybe he was punishing himself for whatever the reason was. It made sense to me then why Steve had always treated me like a daughter. *Maybe he sees me as a second chance*, I thought, *so he's taken me under his wing.* Nonetheless, this man taught me how to fly. He saw me when I felt like no one else did. He showed me how to crank up the resistance when I didn't believe in my own strength.

I shot Steve a contemplative look and did my best to make my eyes say, "I get it." I didn't ask questions, but from that moment on I just understood that this man was as broken as I was. There was this emotional ruthlessness we both shared, which is what made us an unlikely pair, yet so curiously bonded. At the end of the day, sometimes you just need someone to share the fight with.

THE UGLY FACE OF BULIMIA

By 2007, after a full year and a half of hibernating, I felt strong enough to "get back on the horse," so to speak, and return to Purchase. This time, I was accepted into the prestigious Creative Writing conservatory, and was excited to spend my days getting lost in poetry, leaving my little nervous breakdown behind me.

I still pushed myself to socialize, but this time with a little more mindfulness. I made an effort to attend parties and campus events, but to keep my anxiety at bay, I carved out time each day to work out at the campus gym, using every technique I'd learned from Steve. I think I would have admitted then that my obsession with working out was a coping mechanism, but it was better than feeling depressed, and it was better than starving myself, so I let myself have it.

Because I still had a lot of anxiety around eating, I created an "eating agenda" for myself, which consisted of 400 calories, every four hours, four times a day. This worked pretty well for a while: one apple, a slice of whole grain toast, and a hardboiled egg for breakfast; salad with a few strips of chicken and light dressing for lunch; plain yogurt and another piece of fruit for snack; and steamed broccoli and shrimp for dinner. Sure, my daily workouts combined with my measured mealtimes still took up far too much of my brain energy, but again, baby steps. I was better than I had been before.

For a while, I actually succeeded at convincing myself I was a well-adjusted young adult, capable of handling anything that came my way. My classes were going well, I was cultivating new friendships, and as long as I stayed glued to my routine, I felt stable and grounded. But there came a point when the monster within me decided to rear its ugly head again, this time with a different face—the face of bulimia.

It never got to the point where I was throwing up after every meal, but I struggled with binge-and-purge episodes anywhere from a couple of times a month to a couple of times a week for about a year and a half. I did it when I felt stressed. I did it when I felt anxious. I did it when I felt socially incapable. Helpless. Overwhelmed. Alone. In the beginning, nearly *all* my episodes occurred after campus parties or other events involving large crowds, lots of drinking, and unstructured socializing.

Each time I'd force myself to go to a party at the apartment of some new person I just met, the scenario was the same. I'd open the door to the too-loud-to-be-talked-over music, the flashing strobe lights, and the overpowering stench of weed, beer, and bad decisions. Instantaneously, I'd be filled with the same familiar dread I felt in high school when trying to choose a table in the cafeteria, that little voice inside of me forever whispering, *You don't belong here.* Because I was calm and self-contained, people continued to perceive me as mysterious and laid back. They were drawn to me. But I felt like a fraud knowing that ninety percent of my energy always was being put toward concealing my uneasiness.

I was unfulfilled by small talk, discouraged by so many personalities competing for validation and trying to impress one another. Oh, the lies we tell one another. The lies we tell ourselves. We're all just performers living in subjective realities. It makes me wonder how much deconditioning it would actually take for people to tell the truth in every moment and be authentic human beings. How much of a risk would that be? I don't care about your name. I don't care about your major, or your job. What makes you tick? What is your deepest fear? What's something you don't want people to know about you?

My vice was that I smoked as many cigarettes as I could, in part because it gave me an opportunity to step outside every thirty minutes and get away from the noise, but also because there's something calming and ethereal about smoke itself, something that beckons people to speak about deeper, more meaningful things. When I was fortunate enough to land myself in a circle of other smokers, the conversation always went in the direction of soulful confessions and philosophical ponderings. Often, this would be the only part of the entire night that truly fulfilled me.

The 2:00 a.m. walk back to my apartment was always contemplative. Still intoxicated, I'd evaluate the night, my personality, and my entire existence. I'd wonder what moved people to behave the way they did and what inhibited me from ever fully letting go. Was I struggling with anxiety? Or did I have a sixth sense of sorts that made me hyper-vigilant, made everything so ultra-magnified? People usually equate self-consciousness with insecurity, but I think it's possible to be self-conscious simply because you are highly perceptive and uncomfortably aware of the thoughts, feelings, and motives of the people around you. I picked up on everything—I saw through people. And my ability to see more in others made me painfully self-critical about my own thoughts, feelings, and motives. It was exhausting and overwhelming but was it a gift or was it a curse? Without a doubt, I decided, it felt much, much more like a curse.

When I'd finally make it to my campus apartment, after drinking for hours on an empty stomach, I'd feel intrigued by the mysteries of the refrigerator. Its heavy white door was all that separated me from a world of new possibilities—an infinity of flavors and textures and colors, and the exhilarating sense that maybe something could satisfy the hunger I felt in the depths of my being. So, I'd nibble on a piece of grilled chicken, then reach for the peanut butter and swallow a few spoonfuls. Still unsatisfied, I'd pick at a piece of leftover pizza until I'd consumed the entire slice. I'd eat all of my feelings until the guilt rose up in me like a slow, suffocating tar. Then consciousness would set in, the reality of what I had done. At that point, the food was no longer food; it was *poison* inside my body. I worked too hard at the gym and was too disciplined with my eating to allow fifteen minutes of pleasure-seeking to counteract all my effort and hard work. So then I'd fix myself some tincture of vodka and vinegar. I'd pump my stomach muscles and scratch at the back of my throat until the saliva became juicy in my mouth. Then I'd choke up my guts untiI I felt clean again.

Because I shared an apartment with thin walls and three other girls, I was never able to throw up in the bathroom like a "normal" bulimic. Instead, I had to walk down to the nearby parking lot, duck inside the back of my Jeep Cherokee, and cough into a plastic bag until everything was out of me. Or sometimes I'd do it in the woods, surrounded by broken tree branches and cigarette butts, carelessly barbaric. Once the deed was done, I'd return to my apartment with bloodshot eyes and a sour mouth and continue as if nothing had happened. I'll admit making myself barf was by far the vilest thing I have ever done. Then again, it never quite felt like I was the one doing it. It was more like an out-of-body experience, as if I were being possessed by something more powerful than me. I let my body lead me and I just went for the ride.

Now, there's something I have to note here. As vulgar as bulimia may seem, the binging part was in a way positive for me in that it marked a breaking point in my eating disorder. Most certainly, it was a violent phase, and most certainly, I was still completely at odds with myself, still nowhere close to being "healthy." But after years of depriving myself of nourishment, my body was finally saying "No." I could no longer fight nature and win. With each binge, my body was taking back the reins. I was losing control.

Eventually, I started binging and purging even when I wasn't drunk. I believe the first time this happened was the day my parents called me to tell me my childhood dog, Shadow, had died.

"We had to put Shadow down," my mom said with so much love and compassion in her voice. "He didn't feel any pain," she tried to reassure me.

I don't remember if I cried on the phone, but after we hung up, it was like a landslide of emotions pounding down on me. I thought about the day we first brought Shadow home from the animal shelter. My sister and I were in the second grade. We had begged my parents for a puppy for months, and finally we got one. Shadow was wild at first, and we were wild for him. How does time take that vitality away? It's something I've never been able to come to terms with. Once I became a teenager, I stopped giving Shadow attention. For years, I was just doing my thing, and he was just *there*—part of that house, taken for granted. Then, all at once, without warning, I would never have the opportunity to pet him again. I'd never have the opportunity to ignore him again, even if I wanted to, and it made me nauseous to think that things at home would not stay the same forever. Things evolve and change and die when you aren't looking. So I threw up my lunch.

Eventually, purging became something I too often relied on, so I took a stand. I said to myself, *I've got to put my foot down here. I have to stop this.* In an attempt to prevent myself from throwing up, I decided that the next time I binged I would exercise to compensate for the calories instead. I remember negotiating with myself after eating a little too much cereal. *Now you can either throw up or run three laps around the campus loop.* And like a good girl, I chose to run. But halfway into my first lap, the tar began to rise within me. I lost control after that—I found myself ten feet into the woods, scratching at my throat and choking up half-digested clumps of Raisin Bran.

During my junior year of college, I began dating a girl named Danielle. Danielle had an energy about her that was nurturing and easy to be around, which pacified a great need in me for companionship when I was again spiraling out of control.. Her consistent, caring company grounded me. She witnessed me wholly and became the only person I felt comfortable eating around. Because Danielle was petite, I was able to trust her portion sizes as a gauge for my own. Her relationship with food was a model for the way I wanted mine to be. She ate healthy, but wasn't fussy. She trusted her body.

When I eventually confessed to Danielle that I was a once-in-a-while bulimic, she responded with a blend of compassion and tenacity. She cared about me deeply and had patience for every other aspect of my personality, but this, this was not something she was going to tolerate. She made it my obligation to *her* as well as myself that I wouldn't hurt myself anymore. She even gave me an ultimatum and told me that if I continued to make myself throw up, she would leave me. Although it was difficult at first for me to accept Danielle's "tough love" approach toward my struggle,

I knew how strong and irrational the monster was within me. I knew it wasn't going to back down until I found the courage to stop feeding it altogether, and I knew it was going to take being accountable to something beyond myself. So I took on the challenge and decided to try and quit purging cold turkey.

FINDING FREEDOM IN LETTING GO

Shortly after Danielle gave me her ultimatum, I found myself alone in my campus apartment one afternoon with a pint of vanilla frozen yogurt. It was that listless time of day between three and four o'clock, and the playful thought poked at me. *You could eat just a spoonful or two, nothing crazy.* I was okay with that. But could I trust myself to eat a modest few bites and then stop? Surely not. Once my spoon got into the carton, there was no stopping until I was scraping the cardboard bottom. Then, very predictably, the feelings of abandonment, the irreversible guilt, and the unbearable heaviness swept over me like a paralyzing wind. I felt the hot, familiar rush of frustration fill my bloodstream and wanted nothing more than to rid my body of the 500 calories and sixty grams of sugar to make myself pure again.

But instead of obeying the impulse, this time, I paused. I took a few deep breaths to center myself, then paced back and forth for a while, hoping the urge would eventually subside. Then, after a few moments, when I finally accepted I would not be able to shake the feeling on my own, I did something I would have never dreamed of doing before. I asked for help. I called Danielle on her cell phone. By this point, I was in fetal position on the floor, nearly shaking, and when Danielle answered, I explained to her how uncomfortable I felt in my body.

"I really, *really* want to do it," I said. "I know I promised I wouldn't, but I feel crazy. Like I *need* to."

I felt silly knowing Danielle had to leave her class and step out into the hallway to console me. After all, I was twenty-three years old, curled up on the carpet like a helpless infant. However, I realize in hindsight that this was a real breakthrough point, and one of the most courageous things I have ever done. After running from my feelings for years, I made the conscious decision to try a different approach. It marked the beginning of my willingness to lower my guard and to be vulnerable, finally understanding that if I didn't face myself head-on, I'd be my own victim for the rest of my life. And Danielle was as supportive and patient with me as I could have asked for.

When I hung up the phone, I remember staring up at the ceiling for however long—I had no concept of time as the waves of so many oceans washed over me. There was pain, sadness, fear, and other indefinable sensations. I remained on the floor, trembling like a junkie going through withdrawal, until something miraculous happened. I no longer desired to throw up. The simple act of allowing myself to bring awareness to my body and be present with my feelings was enough to liberate me in that moment from years of struggle. No longer did I need to prove anything to anyone, not even myself. I listened to the breath in my lungs. I thought about my heartbeat and all the cells and organs in my body working in perfect, involuntary harmony. I gave myself permission to simply *exist*.

–

My senior year of college, I had trouble sleeping. I'd wake up in the middle of the night, manically inspired with thoughts and ideas. I spent most of that year working to complete my senior poetry portfolio, which I titled *Burying the Butterfly*. In it, I played a lot with the theme of transformation, with butterflies representing the intangible world of thoughts and ideas we tend to chase after. *Burying the Butterfly*, then, was meant to signify my own coming to terms with the reality of things. I was finally ready to be more like the caterpillar, grounded in appreciation for what was right before my eyes. My journey may have been backwards in this way; I learned how to fly before I learned how to crawl. I had to give up my wings to gain back my humanity.

One sleepless night, I happened to be checking my email around three in the morning, and there in my inbox was something addressed to the graduating class of 2009. It was a call for entries for those interested in submitting an essay to be considered for the senior commencement speech. Finalists would be asked to read their essays before a panel of judges, and from there, the senior commencement speaker would be chosen. I remember thinking, *Should I enter?* Then, *Oh, why the hell not? Be spontaneous, Marissa.* And with that, I began typing as fast as I could. I composed an essay on the spot and submitted it within the hour.

To my surprise, I received a response days later informing me I had been chosen as one of the finalists, and that auditions were being held the following afternoon. You'd think I would have thought about what to wear, but somehow it never crossed my mind. Instead, I showed up in bright orange pants and a white button-down shirt covered in intentionally splattered paint. There I was, standing in a formed line of about eight fellow seniors—the girls all dolled up in dresses and updos, and the guys in prim and proper suits. I thought, *Just my luck.*

Nonetheless, I read my speech before the panel with as much conviction as I could muster. I quoted Ralph Waldo Emerson's essay, "Circles," which, though written in the 1800s, rather summed up a lot for me.

> In nature every moment is new; the past is always swallowed and forgotten; the coming only is sacred. Nothing is secure but life, transition, the energizing spirit. No love can be bound by oath or covenant to secure it against a higher love. No truth so sublime but it may be trivial tomorrow in the light of new thoughts. People wish to be settled; only as far as they are unsettled is there any hope for them.

Throughout the essay, Emerson describes the circle as "the highest emblem in the cipher or the world," the primary shape that is inherent in all aspects of nature. He speaks of "the Unattainable, the flying Perfect, around which the hands of man can never meet" to illustrate the illusion that anything in this life can be achieved or attained. That nature is something that "looks provokingly stable and secular, but has a cause like all the rest[...]. There are no fixtures in nature. The universe is fluid and volatile. Permanence is but a word of degrees." According to Emerson, everything new is born out of the ruins of something that existed before. And in every new moment, man has the opportunity to love, aspire, and create new possibilities.

No more than an hour after my audition, my phone rang, and it was one of the judges calling to tell me I had been selected to be the senior commencement speaker for my graduating class. Needless to say, I was ecstatic; not only because I felt validated in my writing and speaking capabilities, but because I had been chosen above everyone else despite showing up to my audition in orange pants and a paint-splattered shirt.

On the day of my graduation, as I read my speech on stage and looked out at the faces of hundreds of people, including my peers, professors, and my family, I reflected on where I had been and where I was going. I thought about the transience of all things and the secrets still incubating inside me. Suddenly it clicked for me what my friend Jen had meant when she told me two years prior that the moon just *is*. There's no such thing as or good or bad, light or dark, or even relativity, really. It's all one big, endless circle, and we're all spiritual just for *being*.

There is no rhyme or reason for why the world turns. There are no standards any of us need to strive for in our lives unless we impose such standards upon ourselves. The moment we stop seeking and accept the present moment is when the moment becomes everything there is. And for the first time, I felt the freedom in this.

PART 2:

10 LIFE TIPS TO HEAL YOU FROM SELF-HARM

I was singing along to one of my favorite songs the other day while driving when the thought occurred to me, *At my core, I'm the exact same person I was when I was nineteen years old.* Sure, I may look older. I do grown-up things now like pay bills and file taxes, but as I belted out the chorus with the speakers turned all the way up, I felt the same emotions in my chest that I'd harbored a decade ago—the yearning to share myself passionately, intensely, and authentically with other people, the desire for freedom and new experiences, and a lustful gratitude for Fiona Apple, who understands me like no real-life person ever has.

There is a pretty miraculous difference though between the person I used to be and the person I am today: I no longer have an eating disorder. And of course, a million things have had to shift in the process of transforming myself from a person who struggles with an illness to a person who does not struggle with an illness. I've put in the work of getting to know myself intimately well. I've created a practice around being present in my body every day, which has enabled me to become more in touch with my truth and more trusting of my decisions. I've decided to embrace the things that make me "odd" or eccentric, rather than judge and punish myself for my perceived limitations.

I've learned to communicate and make choices that make me happy. I've gained self-confidence. And I've homed in on my talents and found ways to share these as gifts with others.

Don't get me wrong; in many ways, even after thirty-one years on this planet, I still don't feel fully adjusted to this world. And yet, I accept all the strangeness. I wake up most days happy and very grateful to be alive. I feed myself nutritious foods. I exercise enough to be healthy but not so much that it's all-consuming and masochistic. I am surrounded by incredible people who love and care about me. I have a job that provides me with lifestyle balance, suits my personality, and aligns with my values. And I live in an apartment in Brooklyn, New York, where I feel stimulated, accepted, and inspired.

If you ask me how to measure progress, I think it must be like this: it's driving alone to your favorite song, feeling compassion for former shades of yourself, but at the same time realizing you're in a whole lot less pain than you used to be. You've evolved into someone wiser. You embrace life as a journey rather than a destination, and you no longer suffer needlessly.

My recovery didn't happen overnight, and my healing journey has been by no means linear. It's been a long, crooked walk complete with relapses and backwards steps. But in the grand scheme of recovering from an eating disorder, even the backwards steps are giant leaps forward, in that they present you with the opportunity to forgive yourself, and to surrender to the inevitable truth that you're not perfect or invincible.

In order to stop feeding the monster that was consuming me, I've had to reallocate that power. I've had to grow up all over again, take responsibility for my own happiness, and find strength in all my shortcomings. This has required knocking down my entire identity and rebuilding it, letting go of previous notions of who I was, allowing rock and rubble to fall where it may, and paving a new path for myself to walk upon this planet. Very gradually, and through a wide variety of healing experiences, I've been able to let go of the idea that I need to hurt myself to save myself.

I'll be the first to admit that what's unknown is often scarier than what's familiar, even when what's familiar is killing you. That is why people remain stuck in abusive relationships and addictions, and it's why I remained stuck for as long as I did. For addicts and people with a fragile sense of who they are, oftentimes continuing to go through the motions of what is familiar is just easier than taking a risk or creating a new opportunity.

While I do believe at least a portion of my eating disorder erupted out of the stereotypical factors that influence many eating disorders—the confusing food climate in America, the body image issues that come with being a woman, etc., I've accepted that the majority of my dysfunctional behaviors around food and exercise were rooted in the fact that I didn't know myself and I was afraid of everything.

As I've continued to seek out the common threads that bind people who have experienced eating disorders, I've come to speculate that eating disorders may occur more frequently in people who are highly sensitive, hypervigilant, and exceptionally attuned with the feelings of the people around them to the point that they feel inclined to protect and nurture others before themselves. They may identify with the term "people pleasers." Carrying on life with such a temperament can be exhausting in that you are constantly absorbing the energy of others, taking on the problems of others, and rarely having an outlet through which to relieve the pressure. And so people like this may be prone to develop eating disorders as a means of controlling the chaos that surrounds them, and to cope with the emotional burden they tend to carry.

I think eating disorders may also occur more frequently in people who are exceptionally driven, perfectionistic, and ambitious, perhaps especially in those who grow up in controlled environments where they are taught to follow many rules, as well as in people who are exceptionally open-minded and inclined toward philosophic thinking.

To create the second half of this book, I've carefully considered how I might break down and simplify everything I've learned in the past ten years into ten life lessons to help others recover from eating disorders, addictions, and other acts of self-harm. Here's what I've come up with:

1. Reflect on the Root Causes of Your Behavior
2. Stop Playing the Victim
3. Make Time to Make Peace with Your Body
4. Speak Up and Ask for What You Need
5. Trust Your Intuition
6. Make Choices That Make You Happy
7. Spend Your Energy Wisely
8. Organize Your Living Space to Promote Wellbeing
9. Eat Mindfully, But Not Neurotically
10. Check in with Yourself as You Evolve

In the following chapters, I'll explain how I arrived at each of these lessons, why I feel passionately about them, and why they are so crucial to health happiness, and general wellbeing. I encourage you to read on with a willingness to consider each of these lessons in the context of your own life. Start thinking about where you are stuck and where you could use support.

Chapter 5
REFLECT ON THE
ROOT CAUSES OF
YOUR BEHAVIOR

-

"Once you realize nothing makes
sense, it all makes sense."
–Unknown

-

Eating disorders thrive on an incredible spectrum of contradictions. I wanted to be in control, but I wanted to surrender control. I wanted to be seen, but I wanted to disappear. It's these and other paradoxes that make eating disorders so difficult to recover from. The abuser is simultaneously the victim.

When I set out to write this book, my ambition was to make *sense* of my experience. I wanted to grab it by the horns like a wild bull, tame it, and present it to you with a neat little bow around it and say, "Here, reader. Now you get it, don't you? Haven't I cracked the code of eating disorders and all of life?" But to my dismay, nothing in this world can be reduced down to such a tidy resolution. Nature is calm, then violent. Fire and water are opposing elements, yet they exist on the same planet, at the same time. So now I have come to accept that there are many thoughts, feelings, and forces that completely contradict one another, and yet they can exist in the same body, at the same time. There is nothing resolved or determined about being a human being; we are never more than complicated processes in motion.

That said, I believe with all my heart in the power of self-awareness. The more we can reflect, meditate, and witness emotions in our bodies, the more consciousness and clarity we bring into our beings. The process of gaining awareness may not *seem* very productive—I mean it's really just being present and reflecting, which may not look like much. But the thing is that awareness leads to action, which leads to experience, which leads to change. I have witnessed this to be true time and time again: when I take the time to be still and meditate on various struggles in my life, I become empowered to take action and do whatever I need to improve a situation. It's almost as if once I connect with my truth, the answers become instantly apparent. And so as a very important first step in my healing journey, I reflected on some of the forces and motives that played a role in the development of my eating disorder. I then compiled the following list:

20 REASONS I STARVED MYSELF

1. **I wanted to express myself.**

   Because I had spent my formative years disentitling myself from being openly expressive at school and in social situations, I was filled with a lot of stifled energy over time. After years of being "quiet," I felt ignored, depleted, and vacant; and because I didn't know how to ask for what I needed verbally, I relied on my body to communicate my inner suffering. I can attest to this: nothing hurts more than pain no one else can see. It was somehow easier to deal with my pain when I made it visible.

2. **I wanted to be in control.**

   I grew up with a lot of rules and in turn felt like I needed to control everything. I was tired of giving my power away to others. I no longer wanted to feel repressed and I no longer wanted to be told what to do. So, I created a reality for myself that only I understood, a reality where I was in charge of the way I felt and could feel.

3. **I wanted to be controlled.**

Here's the first contradiction. Although I was hungry for autonomy, I also craved the safety and familiarity of being disciplined, since I had spent my whole life obeying my parents, teachers, and other authority figures. So I assumed a kind of militant control over my body that simultaneously controlled me.

4. **I wanted to stunt my physical growth and maturation.**

I felt an unprecedented amount of guilt for growing up. My parents were my greatest source of security and comfort, and I was afraid of disappointing them by no longer being dependent on them. I feared puberty. I feared my body becoming anything I wasn't yet prepared to inhabit.

5. **I wanted to protect myself.**

My eating disorder served as a protective barrier between me and other people at a time when I felt especially fragile and overwhelmed. It kept me sheltered inside a bubble that no one could penetrate.

6. I wanted to punish myself.

By not asserting myself in social situations, by not expressing my needs and desires, and by not entitling myself to feel all of my feelings, I let myself down in a really big way. Because of how cowardly and incompetent I allowed myself to appear, I actually started to believe there was something wrong with me, and I wanted to punish myself for being the source of this pain.

7. I wanted to be able to trust myself.

Because I felt incapable of speaking up for myself, I didn't trust myself as someone I could rely on. I was therefore seduced by the sense of personal responsibility that came with disciplining my body, as it gave me the opportunity to "show up" for myself in other ways. Granted, I was showing up for myself only in the areas of extreme dieting and exercise, overcompensating for the areas in which I was lacking. But it still made me feel more confident to know I was capable of setting goals for myself and following through with them.

8. I wanted to be rescued.

It was my deepest hope when I was suffering that someone would have the courage to stop me on the street, peer into my hollow face, and ask me, "Are you okay?" I pushed myself as hard as I could to prove I was invincible, but at the root of it all, I just wanted to be recognized. I wanted someone to "blow my cover," so to speak, to peel back my layers and discover me for my goodness, my pain, and all the weight I was bearing in my fragile heart. I wanted to be taken care of in all the ways I felt unequipped to care for myself.

9. I wanted to be admired.

Because I was not very athletic growing up, it felt good to be admired for my strength and physique, especially at the gym. After a lot of hard work and deprivation, my body became a trophy to me, one I was proud of. I considered myself passionate, even somewhat of a martyr in my mission to rise above my physical appetite, and I wanted others to notice.

10. I wanted companionship.

Sometimes we need to create external worlds, external "love affairs" for ourselves, in order to create a sense of companionship to fill a void we feel inside. I created my eating disorder the way a child might create an imaginary friend, and I don't think it's any coincidence that I relied on it more as I spent less time with my sister and gained more independence from my parents. I craved the consistent company I had always been used to.

11. I wanted revenge.

There's an element to restrictive eating that is passive-aggressive in that the body becomes a quiet, vindictive statement that says, *Look what you made me do to myself.* Because I'd always felt like a bit of an outcast, and because I was painfully shy, I'd allowed others to make me feel inferior, as if my words were less worth saying, as if my thoughts and feelings were less worth expressing, and as if my presence was less worth acknowledging. So I came to identify as a victim in a world of aggressors. I felt justified in blaming my pain on the outside world because I didn't yet know how to take responsibility for it myself. All I knew was that I needed to be validated for the things I had endured.

12. I wanted to feel accomplished / have a purpose / be productive.

I felt strongly that I had a mission in the world, but I had not yet determined what it might be. By preoccupying myself with cautious meal plans and tedious exercise regimens, I was able to feel pseudo-productive even on days when I didn't do much else. My ritualistic habits helped ground me with an artificial sense of purpose, control, and self-sufficiency when I felt otherwise listless and lost.

13. I wanted to test my limits.

When you repress your emotions as often as I did, it creates a dangerously forceful momentum in the body. In my particular case, this momentum became a ruthless determination that enabled me to push my body to virtually superhuman limits. I was already used to denying my own needs so much of the time and just bearing it that it was easy for me to dissociate from my body when it came to tolerating hunger and rigorous exercise. Then, in realizing the unique strength of which I was capable, I became curious about how far I could take it.

14. I wanted to feel contained.

As a contradiction to wanting to feel limitless, I simultaneously wanted to feel contained. I was pushing to find bounds within which I should live, because on a very real level, I needed those parameters. Reality had become too vast, too limitless, so I used dieting to create some order within the chaos. Providing myself a clear path with a simple set of rules to follow pacified my anxiety and made me feel safer.

15. I wanted to feel connected to something beyond the physical world.

After spending my childhood years submerged in Catholicism, I was on a quest to define spirituality on my own terms. Since I was very young I'd been curious about the meaning of life. In my adolescence, I became more existentially focused on the idea that everything is temporary, transient, and ethereal. So when I was experiencing pain in my immediate reality, my instinct was to want to connect to something greater—some divine force that would love me unconditionally and accept me without judgment.

16. I wanted to rebel against the status quo.

In the same way a person might cover themselves in piercings or dye their hair purple, I wanted to stand out from the status quo. I wanted to challenge people's rigid conceptions of the way a young female should look and behave. So what if I was skin and bones and more muscular than most girls? I was rebelling against society's standards and expectations of who and what I should be.

17. I wanted to avoid dealing with my real problems.

There were things about myself I didn't know how to fix, like my social anxiety. So putting all of my energy into food and exercise was very much like procrastinating when you know you have something really difficult to do, like writing a fifteen-page research paper on a subject you don't understand anything about. By projecting all my fears, needs, and desires onto my relationship with food, I was able to avoid dealing with my actual problems.

18. I wanted to eliminate the possibility that I could ever be abandoned.

I had a fear of loss and abandonment which I sought to control through food. Each time I finished a meal, a sort of depression would set in, reminding me of my own mortality. And so on some irrational plane, I figured that if I didn't indulge in anything in the first place, then nothing of value could be taken away from me.

19. I wanted my body to be androgynous.

As a queer person who identifies more with androgyny than femininity, I was afraid of allowing my body to "bloom" into a shape that would not align with the way I felt on the inside. I was comfortable with straight hips and a flat chest. The thought of having boobs, thighs, or curves made me cringe, and I didn't mind losing my period. For many reasons, I have often felt awkward referring to myself as a *woman*.

20. I wanted to stop time.

I felt overwhelmed by the many new responsibilities I was expected to take on before I even had the life experience to understand who I was and what I needed to be happy. I wanted to press "pause" on the speeding world so that I could take some time to turn inward and process it all.

Chapter 6
STOP PLAYING
THE VICTIM

-

"As we are liberated from our own fear, our presence automatically liberates others."
–Marianne Williamson

-

For the entirety of the time I spent sick, I was pushing with as much resistance as possible to avoid having to face the void inside me. But the more I tried to distract myself from the inner work I really needed to be doing, the more intense my fear, pain, shame, and anxiety became, and the crazier I eventually felt. I can acknowledge it now—the reason I refused to face myself is because I was attached to the notion that I was a victim.

On a subconscious level, I'd convinced myself that my eating disorder was a *justified* response to the society within which I lived. It was a valid reaction to the things I'd experienced in my life. "It's not my fault I don't fit in," I thought. "It's not my fault I feel like an outcast most of the time. I am entitled to express myself in this way." I have a right to express myself in this way." After all, I was angry. I held anger toward myself and toward all the people in my life who couldn't read my mind or understand what I was feeling. I felt incapable of relating to others due to my social anxiety and sensitivity. I was in fact so desperate to be validated for the years I had spent feeling powerless and invisible through my years in school, that I was attached to the idea that I had to keep fighting to receive the recognition I deserved. Refusing to see my happiness as my own responsibility, I resented other people for all the things I felt I lacked. I distrusted nearly everyone in my life because I didn't trust myself, and as a result I withdrew violently inward.

As I confessed in the previous chapter, one of my reasons for starving myself was that I wanted to be rescued. I wanted people to feel sorry for me, yet I refused to ask for the help I knew I needed. Instead, I used my body as a pawn in my own passive-aggressive scheme. I figured if I destroyed my body in a way that was visible to others, someone would have to notice and then someone would have to swoop in and save me.

Suffering, as I now see it, is a result of giving in to helplessness. (Some people turn this helplessness into violence against others and some people turn violent against themselves.) It's fear-based. It's deciding to hold onto judgment and hatred. Vibrating at a low energy frequency. Resisting change.

An expression I resonate with now is this: *Where you place your blame is where you place your power.* By placing my blame on the external world, my past, other people, and all the unfair things that had "happened" to me, I gave these people and things the power to control my self-esteem, my self-worth, and my happiness. I created my own prison, never realizing I was holding my own self captive and denying myself the opportunity to heal.

I have since realized that I am responsible for my own happiness, and with this responsibility comes a great deal of power. By no means am I able to prevent myself from experiencing *all* suffering; suffering is a part of life. But what I can do is liberate myself from needless *additional* suffering. I can choose each and every day to be kind, compassionate, patient, and forgiving. I can own the decisions I make and resist blaming others. I can entitle myself to *feel* and witness my emotions without judgment or fear. And I can act to make my life better by taking risks and confronting the things I need to confront. Then as a result of taking good care of myself, I will organically bring more positivity to others.

As a first step to giving up the victim role, I had to actually acknowledge the pain I've gone through and entitle myself to it. Metaphorically speaking, I had to get down on my knees, look former versions of myself in the eye, and say, "What you went through was real. And it sucked. I see you, and I'm here for you." I had to provide the kind of nurturing to myself that I had been waiting for from other people. For my whole life until recently, it's been difficult for me to admit when I'm hurt. I've always had a tendency to undermine my pain and say, "Well, it could be *worse*. Who am I to complain? I come from a good family and I'm lucky to have both a mother and a father. I've never been physically abused, kidnapped, or raped. There are wars going on in the world. I have no right to feel troubled."

But not all trauma is caused by acute traumatic incidents. Sometimes trauma, like the kind I experienced, can be developmental. For example, the years I spent shaking in my skin feeling anxiety-ridden, excluded, trampled over, oppressed, ashamed, lost, lonely, and silenced in the world has had a profound impact on my emotional development and wellbeing over time. So entitling myself to say, "This happened and it hurt me, and it's okay to feel this way," has been a total game-changer.

Another important piece of this is understanding that not every feeling you have is going to seem rational, warranted, or fair to other people, but that doesn't make those feelings illegitimate. It doesn't invalidate them or eliminate your need to experience them for what they are. We all live in subjective realities, after all, where our experiences may be magnified or distorted depending on a number of factors. Some of these factors include: age and level of experience (children often have very different emotional reactions to things than adults do, based on their limited life experience); emotional temperament (sensitive people may experience emotions and sensations more vividly than non-sensitive people); and mental health (people who suffer with certain mental health issues may have magnified experiences and magnified reactions to those experiences based on their specifically altered sense of reality).

I accept now that there is light and dark inside of every human being and that the most evolved people are not those who have less darkness, but rather those who have mastered the art of co-existing with their darkness. When one is trying to deny the darkness, escape it, or repress it as I did is when that darkness will cast a black shadow over your entire life. And that shadow can move a person to do all kinds of crazy things. This is why it's so important we look our demons in the eye and confront them. Whatever has happened to you in the past and whatever cards you have been dealt in this life—maybe it's not your fault, but it's still your responsibility to heal your own scars and nurture yourself to become the person you want to be.

Chapter 7
MAKE TIME TO MAKE
PEACE WITH YOUR BODY

-

The body can be a strange thing. Essentially, the body is a random animal we inhabit for the time we spend on this earth. We don't choose our race, our gender, our sexuality, or if we'll have smile lines by the time we're thirty. Some people feel disconnected from their bodies. Some feel insecure about the shape of their nose or the size of their thighs or the freckles on their skin. Some feel limited by their physical capacities. And some feel as if they were born into the wrong body altogether.

Throughout my eating disorder, I experienced a great sense of dissociation from my body, meaning I did not identify with it. Instead, I felt more like there was a "me" which was my mind, operating my body as if it were a piece of machinery. The year after I graduated college, I did some nude modeling for the art classes at Purchase and stripped myself naked in front of my peers for fifteen dollars an hour. I held poses upon a raised platform, remaining completely still in each position, sometimes for twenty minutes or more.

In making the decision to do nude modeling, there were both positive and negative motives at play. On one hand, I thought posing nude might provide me an opportunity to become more comfortable in my body through being so vulnerably exposed. But admittedly, the not-fully-recovered part of me was entranced by the idea of a roomful of budding artists admiring my naked, androgynous body. It isn't a thing most people get to experience—being studied intently by twenty people at once while listening to the choir of twenty pencils scratching your form onto paper, validating your existence.

Sometimes the instructor would refer to me as "the model," or "the subject." He was careful never to use my name, as if doing so would break some forbidden fourth wall; as if doing so would suddenly "out" me to everyone in the room as a human being with thoughts and fears and feelings, making it unbearably awkward for me to be standing bareass naked on a pedestal. So in the name of keeping things professional, I was totally objectified. And that felt okay at the time, because my body was only a costume I was wearing. I was even entertained by the notion that I could exist somewhere in my head, protected from the entire experience, concealed even when I should be most visible.

Today, the way I feel about my body is entirely different; my body is a part of me. I'm not sure I could so comfortably strip for a roomful of strangers in the present day—not because I feel shame and not because I am uncomfortable in my skin, but because I feel my own body to be something sacred and worth protecting. I've come to understand that the relationship I have with my body is the most important relationship I'll ever have. Imagine being stuck in an elevator with one person for your entire life—your body is that person. And so whether or not you completely jive with everything God gave you, you sure as hell better find a way to get along with your body like it's your best friend. If you don't, there will always be consequences.

So how did I go from feeling totally detached from my body to wholly embracing it? Well, it took bearing a lot of discomfort at first. But in time I discovered the importance of making time to be present in my body. Simply existing inside of my skin consciously and intentionally has enabled me to access the profound and mysterious intelligence that each of our bodies hold. Your body is in fact wiser than you will ever be. It knows how much food you need and sends you signals to let you know when you're full. It knows when you're tired and sends you signals that it's time to rest. It knows when you're injured and sends you signals in the form of pain. Sometimes I remind myself of all the systems and processes that are occurring in my body in every moment to keep me alive and I feel an overwhelming sense of gratitude.

That said, the most profound healing for me has occurred in the act of consciously inhabiting my body and witnessing my emotions when it's been the least comfortable for me to do so. Often, people's first instinct is to ignore or escape negative feelings. They'll seek out a distraction to preoccupy their minds from having to confront sadness, anxiety, or pain. Or they'll attempt to numb their feelings with a substance like alcohol or drugs (or food). But what I've found to be true is something Carl Jung said: "What you resist, persists." When you run from your fears and insecurities, they never go away. They in fact just get bigger and bigger.

Alternatively, when you choose to witness your negative emotions without judgment and without the intent to control them, you disempower them. I like to think of it as "bearing the ice bath." Inhabiting the body when you most feel like escaping it is uncomfortable, of course, but it's transformative. I'll go to the extent of trying to force myself right into the belly of the pain. For example, if I'm going through a breakup, I might carve out some intentional time in my day to listen to evocative music while going through pictures of the person I am losing. This experience might move me to tears, and if it does, I will allow myself to cry until I am done crying. Sometimes I'll incorporate some journaling so I can witness my emotions on paper and follow them to their source. The miracle is that by approaching my feelings with tolerance rather than resistance, I prevent those emotions from taking me over. Pain eventually dissipates like a passing storm.

–

Something else I want to address in this chapter is gender identity and sexuality since I have personally encountered an overlap between eating disorders, dissociative disorder, and gender dysphoria. Let's begin by defining gender dysphoria; this term refers to an extreme discomfort with one's body based on the biological sex one is born into. Oftentimes people who experience gender dysphoria feel that their emotional and psychological identity does not align with the gender they were assigned at birth.

One driving force behind my eating disorder was that I wanted my body to appear more androgynous. Small boobs, straight hips, and a scrawny yet toned body was my ideal (think Shane from *The L Word*). So for me the incentive to be skinny was driven by more than a resistance toward being "fat." It was also driven by my resistance to being a "woman." I knew if I gained even a few pounds, those pounds would go straight to my hips and thighs and make me appear overtly more feminine. So my gender identity was at stake along with everything else. It's not that I wanted to be a man, necessarily. But I did want to challenge the social expectations that came with inhabiting my female body.

This was my form of gender dysphoria. Long before I even knew I was a lesbian, I just wasn't into embodying society's idea of "what a girl should be." I never wanted to wear dresses or paint my nails. As a child, I preferred playing with "boy" toys like Ninja

Turtles, dinosaurs, and matchbox cars. Then as a teenager, I never got into makeup or felt attracted to boys in magazines. In an attempt to "fit in," I followed the cues of other girls and did what I thought I was "supposed" to do—I plastered my walls with pictures of N'Sync, the Backstreet Boys, and Freddie Prinze, Jr., but none of it ever came naturally. By the eleventh grade, when I realized I was a girl attracted to girls in a world where everyone else seemed straight or at least pretended to be, it was partially a relief, because everything finally made sense. But in other ways, I felt even more like an outcast and internalized some shame around my body and my preferences. I developed a skewed sense of self-worth coming of age in a society that didn't seem to have a place for me.

Now let's return to my theory that people who experience gender dysphoria are more likely to develop an eating disorder. This makes sense to me since gender dysphoria often includes elements of dissociation, and dissociation is a common trait of eating disorder sufferers. Aspects of dissociation include a lack of connection with the body, the emotions, the authentic self, the community, the world, and a higher purpose and meaning in life.[3]

Whether related to gender or something else, this dissociative aspect of eating disorders is important to recognize. If a person does not identify with their body, they are going to have a greater propensity toward self-harm, or at the very least they may be drawn to experiment with their body in a quest to gain perspective and understand what is real.

Now, when it comes to gender dysphoria, I don't think we can consider one's level of discomfort with the body they are born into without also considering what we have been conditioned to believe about men vs. women. When a person feels uncomfortable in the gender they are born into, is it actually their gender that they feel they don't identify with? Or is it that they don't identify with the roles, expectations, and ideals that society has *assigned* to that gender? It's unfortunate but true; social conditioning intrudes on many aspects of our developing selves and plays a significant role in the way we come to conceive of ourselves in the world. We are conditioned to believe

---

3. Kobrin, Shoshana, MA, LMFT. "Dissociation and Eating Disorders: Restoring the Shattered Shards." The International Association Of Eating Disorders Professionals Foundation. https://iaedp.confex.com/ iaedp/2014/ webprogram/Session2486.html (accessed 2017).

we *should* be so many things considered to be the ideal, then we're taught to measure ourselves against these ideals and determine our self-worth accordingly. So when groups of people rebel in their bodies through eating disorders or other means, I think it's worth examining society's role in this behavior, and to what degree the behavior may be a form of acting out in response to standards perceived to be unfair or exclusionary.

Unfortunately, there are many reasons a person might be driven to resist the idea of being a woman. Throughout history and in most cultures, women have been forced into submissive and secondary roles as compared to men. Women have had to fight for rights, equality, and power, whereas it seems that for men, these things have always been their birthright. Even in the modern day, there is a level of gender conditioning that begins in childhood—toys made for boys include fierce-looking figurines, GI Joes, video games, and plastic weapons, as if to prepare them to become superheroes; whereas girls get toy cooking sets, dolls, and toy baby strollers as if to prepare them for a future in caretaking and homemaking. In adolescence, girls learn that wearing makeup and fashionable clothing will make them popular, whereas for boys, it's more about alpha confidence and being good at sports. And finally, as adults society teaches us that a successful woman is one who "has it all together"—one who can pop out babies and be a good mother while maintaining a career while maintaining her looks and body at the same time. Social standards for men seem to revolve more around the amount of money they earn and the amount of power they have. So when I think of the word *woman* through the lens of my conditioning, I am uncomfortable. I don't want to be obedient, passive, accommodating, needy, or weak, all words I have been brainwashed to think of when I see a female figure reflected at me in a mirror.

Maybe you're not someone who feels a sense of gender dysphoria but you still experience dissociation from your body as a result of inhabiting a body that is not celebrated by the world around you. Perhaps you don't identify with your ethnicity. Or maybe your feelings of dissociation have nothing to do with your outward appearance. Maybe you feel a level of discomfort in your skin because you are gay or introverted or disabled. I think it's worth hypothesizing that minorities of any kind are more likely to have a lowered sense of self-worth and self-confidence than non-minorities. They are more prone to self-doubt, self-hate, and self-harm in that they are consistently exiled by a world that does not offer them inclusion or representation. Moreover, minorities, especially members of the lesbian, gay, bisexual, transgender and questioning and others (LGBTQ+) community, are more frequently targeted as victims of hate crimes; they're more discriminated against and more likely to be ostracized even by their own families.

Now I will say that we've made a good amount of progress as a society in the past couple of decades, but when I entered adolescence at the turn of the millennium, it was a much different world. The Internet was only just beginning to emerge, so there was no such thing as YouTube, which has become a platform for young people around the world to share progressive ideas on many topics, including sexuality. The LGBTQ+ community had very little representation in the media; shows like *The Ellen DeGeneres Show* and *The L Word* didn't premiere until the year I graduated high school. Social media was only just beginning to become a thing. So until the age of eighteen or so, I had virtually no role models who were gay. I had very few examples of "alternative" lifestyles to aspire toward and very limited resources available to me.

Thankfully, today, at least here in America, the generation coming of age is beginning to acknowledge the many variations in gender and sexuality in ways that are more inclusive to people who feel other than "straight." You may have heard of terms like "non-binary," which describes any gender identity that does not fit into the male and female binary.[4] In this case, the binary refers to the system of viewing gender as consisting solely of two identities and sexes, man and woman or male and female. Other terms being used include "agender," which refers to people whose gender identity and expression does not align with man, woman, or any other gender; "bigender," which refers to someone whose gender identity encompasses both man and woman; "gender fluid," "gender non-conforming," "genderqueer," etc. By now, most people are familiar with the term "transgender," which is an umbrella term for people whose gender identity and/or expression is different from cultural and social expectations based on the sex they were assigned at birth.[5] By the way, these terms point only to gender

---

4. "Non-binary." Gender Wiki. http://gender.wikia.com/wiki/Non-binary (accessed 2017).

5. Adams, Cydney. "The gender identity terms you need to know." CBS News. https://www.cbsnews.com/news/transgender-gender-identity-terms-glossary/ (accessed 2017).

identity. There are also a slew of available terms to describe sexuality, which is not necessarily correlated with gender identity. For example, a transgender woman who is attracted only to women may choose to identify as a lesbian. How one defines oneself in terms of gender identity should not imply anything about who one should be attracted to.

Unfortunately, for some people these concepts are going to take time to understand. The other day, for example, I found myself in a conversation about sexuality with two women my age who identify as straight. One of the women actually shocked me with her arrogance when speaking about gender roles in same sex partnerships.

"I just don't understand why some girls make themselves look like guys and why other girls are attracted to that," she said. "I saw a lesbian couple at the airport the other day and this one girl looked like a total dude. I just don't get it. Like why not just be with a dude."

In response, I did my best to keep my cool and educate her. I reminded her that sexuality is very layered and complex, as is attraction. Some people are attracted to masculinity in women but *not* masculinity in men. I think our culture has this current fascination with people who identify anywhere on the LGBTQ+ spectrum because the idea of gender and sexuality existing on a spectrum is still a rather new concept for some. People are intrigued but also judgmental, because they fear what they don't understand. My feeling is that we are putting too much responsibility on the LGBTQ+ community to make "alternative" relationships and "alternative" sex acts more acceptable and mainstream. The thing is, the complexities behind the way people feel about themselves and what turns people on are not exclusive to the LGBTQ+ community—these things are very layered and complicated for people who identify as straight as well. For example, I read somewhere recently that a surprisingly high percentage of women fantasize about being gangbanged when they're having sex. However, the number of women who would actually want to experience a gangbang is much, much smaller. Some people have foot fetishes. Some like to be peed on. So why is it so difficult to understand a woman being attracted to another woman who dresses in "men's" clothing? I myself have a very difficult time understanding heterosexual relationships since I have never experienced being attracted to a man, and yet I have no choice but to accept these relationships, because they're around me every day, every time I turn on the TV, everywhere I go. I don't have the "privilege" of debating the legitimacy of heterosexual relationships because they're considered mainstream and I am the minority.

The bottom line is that I don't think it's anyone's place to judge what another person likes or dislikes, whether or not they understand it. Everyone should have the right to love, fuck, and express themselves freely, regardless of what body they are born into. At the end of the day, you don't have to "get it," you just have to accept it. There is no greater human virtue than having tolerance for the things we don't understand. And this tolerance begins with ourselves.

That said, I don't think we're at a point yet in society's evolution where we can consider gender identity without also considering the ways in which we've been socially conditioned and thereby affected by various ideals of what gender should and shouldn't be. However, for the sake of future generations, I do hope that they are burdened by fewer of these expectations and given the opportunity from birth to inhabit the bodies they are born into without preconceived notions of what their sexual organs should imply.

In the meantime, all we can do is work to gain as much self-awareness as possible of the ways in which we've been socially conditioned, and we can try to decondition ourselves as much as possible. But realistically speaking, we cannot totally and completely reverse all the social conditioning we've been subject to our entire lives. Whether we are to some extent conforming to social ideals or rebelling against them, we are still propelled by these ideals, and at some point all we can do is accept this.

To this day I still prefer to exist in a body that is as close to androgynous as I can maintain—I feel at peace with my body and in alignment with my gender identity when I am thin with a little bit of muscle tone, and I am grateful I've been able to maintain this kind of body for many years now without depriving myself. My goal is no longer to be scrawny or malnourished: I work out and eat mindfully to feel good about myself. It's still part of my self-expression, just in a healthier way.

Now you might be thinking, "I thought this chapter was about tolerance, acceptance, and finding peace inside the body you have—not changing your body to fit your idea of who or what you should be." My answer to this is that it's a little bit of both. I fully support using the mind to see beyond the physical realm and transcend the body in a spiritual way through meditation, etc., but we are spiritual beings in a material world. I'm not going to tell you your appearance won't matter while you're here. People will judge you based on the way you look, and that is just a fact of life. That is not to say you should allow anyone else to place expectations on you in terms of the way you *should* look or feel in your body. But I do think you deserve to reside in a body you feel good about—a body that aligns with the way you feel on the inside. And so I do encourage you to set realistic goals for yourself and do whatever it is you need to do to become the best version of you. Then surrender to the rest. Ask yourself, "What is the home I would feel most comfortable in?" Then, "What is within my power in terms of achieving this home for myself, and what is not within my power? Am I willing to push myself to change the things I can change, and am I willing to love and accept myself for the things I cannot change?"

When you're able to master the balance between striving to be better and accepting yourself for where you presently are…when you're able to comfortably inhabit your body despite social conditioning, ideals, and expectations…and when you're able to withstand the "ice bath" of your own emotions for long enough to make peace with your own darkness, you will naturally begin to operate from a place in your heart that does not judge or criticize others, and you will contribute to making the world a better place just by existing as you are.

Chapter 8
SPEAK UP AND ASK FOR WHAT YOU NEED

-

"Most people believe vulnerability is weakness. But really, vulnerability is courage. We must ask ourselves...are we willing to show up and be seen?"

—Brené Brown

-

My favorite scene in the movie *Fight Club* is when Brad Pitt's character, Tyler, and Edward Norton's character (who is never officially named, but we'll call him Jack) are standing outside a bar after drinking three pitchers of beer together. Jack's apartment unit has just been torched in a fire, so he's lost all his possessions and has no place to stay. Their dialogue goes like this:

JACK. I should find a hotel.

TYLER. What? A hotel?

JACK. Yeah.

TYLER. Just ask, man.

JACK. What are you talking about?

TYLER. [Laughs] Three pitchers of beer and you still can't ask.

JACK. What?

TYLER. You called me 'cause you needed a place to stay.

JACK. Oh hey, no, no.

TYLER. Yes, you did. So just ask, cut the foreplay. Just ask, man.

JACK. Would that be a problem?

TYLER. Is it a problem for you to ask?

JACK. Can I stay at your place?

TYLER. Yeah.

JACK. Thanks.

What makes this scene in the movie is that Jack is clearly someone who is depressed, in search of meaning. His character wrestles with the humdrum monotony and facades that are part of his daily routine and modern society. Yet he plays into it. He chooses, perhaps unconsciously, to beat around the bush rather than asking Tyler clearly and directly right off, "Would it be okay if I stayed with you for a while?"

As human beings, or at least as Americans, I'm not sure why so many of us automatically disguise our wants, needs, and desires rather than permitting ourselves to say what we really mean. Are we afraid that asking for what we want will make us too vulnerable? Are we afraid of putting other people on the spot? Of being impolite? Women tend to struggle with this even more than men in that we have been more conditioned to put others' needs before our own. We've also been taught to avoid conflict, to please the people around us, and to maintain the peace, sometimes without regard for own sanity or wellbeing.

In the context of my eating disorder, this notion of feeling afraid to assert my desires manifested as a fear of my own appetite. I didn't want to be hungry for anything because I saw hunger as a weakness and as vulnerability. To be able to say, "I'm hungry to be...treated with respect, taken care of, touched, desired, listened to," was petrifying, as I had come to believe that having an appetite for anything was something to be ashamed of. Since I was afraid to speak up for myself, I simply went along with the things that others expected of me. I avoided every opportunity to put myself out there and be seen. I was basically a passenger on the train of my own life—all my friendships and relationships were with people who pursued me, as I never had the guts to approach people I was interested in. I was so terrified of rejection, I could never bring myself to make the first move, whether that meant initiating a conversation with a stranger or initiating intimacy with a lover. I chose self-preservation instead.

In a very popular TED talk called *The Power of Vulnerability*, researcher-storyteller Brené Brown states that connection is why we're here. It's what gives purpose and meaning to our lives. She goes on to describe the years she spent studying vulnerability and how she arrived at a conclusion: there are two kinds of people—people who have a strong sense of love and belonging and people who don't. The one variable that separates the one group from the other is worthiness. Some people feel worthy of love and connection and some don't. Brené's work led her to identify a few commonalities among the group of people she refers to as "whole-hearted." They had the courage to be imperfect; they had compassion toward

themselves and others; they were able to let go of who
they thought they should be in order to be who they
authentically were, and they embraced vulnerability as
essential. According to Brené, vulnerability is the core
of shame and fear and of our struggle for worthiness,
but it's also the birthplace of joy, creativity, belonging,
and love. As a final point in her talk, Brené asserts that
we cannot selectively numb emotions, meaning that
we can't choose to block out negative emotions while
still feeling positive emotions; either we're feeling
everything, or we're numbing ourselves from pain
as well as joy, gratitude, and happiness. And when
we're numb, we're segregated from our purpose
and meaning.

One of the biggest life lessons I've had to learn is
how to stand up for myself and how to communicate
my needs to others. This is in fact the complete
opposite of being passive-aggressive—waiting for
others to notice what you need and punishing them
when they don't. While I still strive to be even more
shamelessly expressive, vulnerable, and authentic, I
have learned that I have an obligation to my own self-
worth. By allowing myself to take risks and be seen
for who I am, I create opportunities for connection
with others. And the more I demonstrate value and

respect myself, the more respect I earn from the people around me. There is in fact a special kind of humbleness in allowing others to see my hunger, my desires, and my humanity. It's intimate—having the courage to be witnessed as we are, wanting what we want, needing what we need. To be vulnerable is to be alive.

Chapter 9
Trust Your Intuition

-

"To know thyself is the beginning of wisdom."
–Socrates

-

One of the great dangers of my personality is that I've always had a tendency to over-challenge my instincts. I think a lot of people operate on impulse— they just feel something and they go with it. In theory, it sounds great to be this free-spirited, in that such people are never stuck in their heads, though they can usually benefit from applying more thoughtful strategy to their lives. Then there are people who move though life with an appropriate amount of self-awareness, grounded in who they are while also conscious of how their words and actions affect others. And then there are people like me. I overcomplicate everything. I weigh every possibility within every situation before acting. And I get stuck in my head. I'm very thoughtful and methodical in the way I do almost everything.

I know it now—the number one reason I suffered from an eating disorder is because I didn't trust my body or myself. As a blooming young adult, I had no sense of my own intuition. Before I reached a point where I felt secure within myself and my identity, I began challenging the ways in which I'd been conditioned. When I knew I felt sexually attracted to women, I said to myself, *Yes, I feel this way. But is this [being gay] my identity? Or am I just emotionally undeveloped in understanding how to connect with men? If I work this out in therapy, will it change?* When it came to being an introvert and feeling like I needed more alone time than other people, I asked more questions. *Is this my actual temperament? Or is it just anxiety? Other people don't seem to feel this way, so why should I?* So I pushed myself to go out and interact with people much more frequently than I felt comfortable doing. I used reason and philosophy to disempower my needs, my desires, and all of my gut feelings.

Time and again I gave myself over to the agendas of those around me; I even allowed others to take advantage of me and then found ways to rationalize their behavior. I've gone to great lengths to protect other people's feelings and reputations—for some reason, that has always felt like an inherent responsibility to me, even at the expense of my own piece of mind. It's no wonder I eventually reached a breaking point. By the time my eating disorder finally erupted, my body was overflowing with years of harbored resentment about all the parts of myself I had given away to others. And even then, I didn't know how to take it out on anyone but myself.

I spent so many years caught up in the external world, relying on other people and things to define me and provide me with a sense of purpose. So it was awkward at first when I finally decided to journey inward and asked myself the question, *What do I want?* As it turns out, no matter how many personality quizzes I take, how many astrology books I read, or how many labels I decide to apply to myself, there is no person or thing "out there" that can really define me. The knowing I have been searching for has come only through the patient process of building trust in my body and myself.

In order to do this, I had to first let go of my preconceived notion that there's something wrong with me or that I am inadequate. I had to accept that I don't need to enjoy the same things other people enjoy to be a legitimate human being. Then I had to journey inward and get to know myself from the inside out. This enabled me to develop self-love and become motivated to nurture myself.

Nowadays my body and I are best friends. Because I have done the work to build a relationship of trust with myself, life is just a whole lot easier now. When it comes to people, I don't have to think so hard anymore about who I should spend time with—I can feel the energy of the people around me, and I'm attuned enough with my own self to know which energies I want to be surrounded by and which energies I don't want anywhere near me. When it comes to social obligations and opportunities, I now recognize my own energy levels and I make an effort not to overcommit myself. That is, I know I am a person who needs time alone each week to recharge, and so I make an effort to carve out that time for myself. I have a lot of friends with whom I love spending time, but I try not to make plans with anyone unless my own needs have been met first. I also make an effort to partake in activities I actually enjoy doing with people, such as having meaningful conversations, cooking, or doing something active like biking or skating. I usually end up feeling drained and overstimulated whenever I push myself to go to crowded bars or clubs, so I try to avoid highly stimulating environments of those kinds. Taking care of myself in these ways helps me to feel more sane and grounded. And when I feel centered and happy, I'm actually a lot more fun to be around.

Chapter 10
MAKE CHOICES THAT
MAKE YOU HAPPY

-

Four years ago, I was working forty hours a week in the busiest part of Manhattan, plus commuting to work nearly an hour each way on a crowded rush hour subway. I was in a volatile relationship that was frequently explosive, and I was living in Brooklyn with no car and no means of escape. Needless to say, I felt claustrophobic and overwhelmed. I was constantly sick, fatigued, and irritable, and it became more evident to me with each passing day that the life I was living was not in alignment with what I deep down wanted for myself.

Then one day I decided to change everything all at once. I quit my job in New York City, I ended my dysfunctional relationship, and I moved to the suburbs where I'd be surrounded by more nature and less hustle and bustle. In deciding to take this leap of faith, everything I wanted lined up for me; I found a great apartment I could afford on my own, I got an opportunity to work from home, and I began dating someone I was genuinely excited about.

Inside my newly flexible lifestyle, I had the rare opportunity to indulge in taking care of myself every single day. I slept eight hours a night and rarely woke to the sound of an alarm. I exercised any time I felt I needed some endorphins. I was able to shop for fresh ingredients and cook healthy meals. I even had the time for all of those girly personal maintenance tasks like shaving my entire body in the shower and using Bioré pore strips. Perhaps most notably of all, I finally had the room in my life to get lost in the patient process of writing this book.

This period was pivotal in that it confirmed the things I need in order to thrive. I need to nurture my body—this includes eating healthy, exercising regularly, sleeping adequately, and occasionally pampering myself; I need time alone to rest, reflect, and recharge—I'm not one of those people who can just keep going; I need the freedom to expand into my creativity; I need the company of loving, supportive people who show up for me emotionally and stimulate my mind; and I need to maintain an open kind of self-awareness as I continue to experiment and grow.

It was through experiencing the contrast between a lifestyle that didn't work for me and a lifestyle that did that I started to take balance a whole lot more seriously. Once I experienced how much happier I could be by doing the things I wanted to do and living my life the ways I wanted to live it, there was no going back. To this day, I'm enjoying the luxury of working from home, which suits my personality and provides me with the time and energy to also focus on passion projects and create a life for myself outside of work.

What it all boils down to is that there is no blueprint for how anyone is supposed to live. It's up to you to get to know yourself and what kind of life is going to make you most happy. Do you want to live in the city, the country, or the suburbs, or maybe on a private island? Do you want to be in a relationship with one person or do you want to be polyamorous? What do you want your career to look like? Do you want to work a nine-to-five or do you want to be your own boss? Then it's up to you to take all the necessary actions to make it happen. The reason most people stay stuck is because they are afraid of taking a risk. But more often than not, when you take a risk in the name of moving yourself into alignment with your truth, the Universe will have your back.

The other part of making choices that make you happy is that you have to stop giving a fuck about what other people think. Because I've felt different from the people around me my whole life, I've struggled a lot with my own self-worth. I was an introvert in a world dominated by extroverts, therefore I thought there must be something *wrong* with me. I hated parties, loud music, and dancing, whereas others seem to be ignited by such environments, therefore there must be something *wrong* with me; I questioned everything in a world where others seemed complacent within the status quo, therefore I was definitely an outcast. And the list went on, the core belief being that "I'm different, therefore I'm *wrong*."

Then one day a light bulb went off and I asked myself, *What if there's nothing wrong with me? What if I didn't judge myself against so many standards of who and what I should be? Would my problems still feel like problems then? Or is my biggest issue that I don't accept myself?*

This got me thinking about all the ways in which I'd been holding myself back because of my own internalized shame and fear around the ways other people perceived me. I finally asked myself: how much time have I wasted paralyzed by self-consciousness? How much energy have I expended trying to fit my behavior, appearance, and personality into various molds? And what if I'm the only one standing in the way of my own happiness? When we hate things in ourselves, we give those things power and we lose the ability to change them. It's only through making the conscious effort to approach ourselves with loving acceptance that we unlock the gate to our own happiness.

Now that I'm an adult I can appreciate my uniqueness and find purpose in it. I can also understand that no matter what I do, there are going to be people who have opinions about it. I simply can't let their opinions get under my skin. Every person born on this planet is born with an equal amount of agency over his or her own life. Nobody knows better than you what's right for you (unless perhaps you are a child or someone who struggles with a severe mental illness or disability). So be bold, take risks, and give yourself the opportunity to grow.

It's been a process that's taken years, but slowly and surely I've been permitting myself to exist in ways that make sense and feel comfortable to me regardless of what others expect. I've found spaces to go where I feel accepted. I've cultivated friendships with people who understand me. I've done my best to create a lifestyle for myself that nurtures my truest nature. And I've decided to give a fuck only when it's actually important to me to give one.

Chapter 11
SPEND YOUR
ENERGY WISELY

—

As I have discovered, creating space in my life for the things that fulfill me is much less about making *time* for these things and much more about budgeting my energy. People often talk about budgeting their money or budgeting their time, but few people talk about budgeting their energy. I like to treat my energy like a bank account; it's renewable but not limitless; I need to replenish it as often as I withdraw from it. Energy is a currency, and it's the most important currency there is.

The majority of us can benefit from being more aware of the fact that different tasks and activities carry different amounts of *energetic weight* in our minds and bodies. Just as a calorie of fat is not the same as a calorie of protein, a minute spent doing something you hate is going to have a different energetic effect on your body than a minute spent doing something you love, regardless of how much time you have left over. So we may as well focus our energy on things that inspire and replenish us—things that are in alignment with who we are and what we care about.

In this chapter, I'm going to focus on five golden rules I feel most passionately about when it comes to spending energy wisely: (1) stop trying to please everyone; (2) choose friends and romantic partners who accept you for you; (3) limit exposure to environments and personalities that drain you; (4) align your everyday work with your personality; (5) and exercise just enough but not too much.

STOP TRYING TO PLEASE EVERYONE

The first golden rule of budgeting your energy has to do with not giving too much of it away to other people. I've already mentioned I've had a lot of difficulty in my life when it comes to setting boundaries and protecting my time and resources. I'm an inherently giving person, plus I've always had a hard time saying no, so as a result, I have had a long history of giving more energetically to the people around me than I could afford. This has led me at various points to become irritable, withdrawn, resentful, and even depressed. I'm not particularly fond of the word *limitations* in reference to what I am able to give. However, I recognize that I have an important responsibility to protect my energy (as much as is possible) from draining personalities, unnecessary obligations, etc, so that I have more of it to distribute to the people and things I truly care about.

When operating from a place of authenticity, I am less likely to lash out at the people around me. I don't carry around a feeling that "the world owes me" because I'm conscious and I'm in control of my own decisions. I'm not saying I never compromise for other people or that I avoid all uncomfortable situations. We all have to compromise every once in a while in order to make relationships work, and we all need to challenge ourselves to take risks and have new experiences in our lives. I'm just saying I do my best to be mindful. And when I move forward with this kind of awareness, I feel like I'm *living*, really *living*, rather than just going through the motions. I'm able to make room for new possibilities and invest more of myself into people and experiences that align with my most authentic self.

I'll admit I still have a bit of a hang-up when it comes to letting other people down. But I try to remind myself that if a person truly loves me, they will trust the boundaries I set for myself and love me beyond their own needs. There is no person's needs on this planet I am capable of meeting one hundred percent of the time. I can only do my best. Running myself into a state of exhaustion trying to be everything to everyone is not going to make me happier, and it's not going to make the world a better place. It's my job to carve out space for myself to exist in the ways I need to exist, even when others won't. And I remind myself daily that those who are meant to be in my life will accept that. I am not selfish for honoring my own needs. Other people's reactions to my boundaries don't determine the validity of my boundaries. And the only thing I need to be one hundred percent of the time is true to myself.

CHOOSE FRIENDS AND ROMANTIC PARTNERS WHO ACCEPT YOU FOR YOU

I try to surround myself with people who align with my values, people who support me, and people who accept me for who I am. Don't get me wrong,

I love being challenged too, and I think some of my most valuable relationships are those that inspire me to grow and become a better person. But there is a healthy balance to be had here. I thrive most when I'm challenged just enough; I like being around people who accept me for who I am when I'm operating from a place of self-love, but who also open me up to new ideas and possibilities. The more I treat myself in ways that are loving, the more I notice the effect this has on the people around me, and the clearer I get on the kinds of people I want to be around.

Now when it comes to romantic relationships, lines tend to get more blurred in terms of healthy boundaries (or maybe I'm just speaking from my own experience). One of the most beautiful things about committing to another person in a romantic relationship is that you get to learn the art of compromise. You get to know what your partner needs, wants, values, etc. And from there you (hopefully) make an effort to meet your partner halfway in terms of your efforts and investment. Most people tend to be a bit more giving when it comes to their romantic partners than they are with their friends. Some even put romantic love on such a pedestal that they put all their partner's needs above their own. This kind of relationship can be described as codependent, and I've been involved in a few codependent relationships myself. Why do some people allow themselves to become so consumed? Well, there are plenty of reasons. Some people are insecure, and they look to their lover to provide them with a sense of purpose. Some people are afraid they'll lose their partner if they don't fill all their partner's needs and expectations. Some people will do whatever they can to avoid conflict and maintain peace.

It is also worth mentioning that I think the media tends to depict true love as this all-consuming force that *should* take us over and inspire us to sacrifice everything, including in some cases even our own lives (*Romeo and Juliet*). Don't get me wrong, I cried at *The Notebook*, just as I'm sure you did too. Selfless love can be beautiful. The problem is I think too many people look for the kind of love that takes them over like a drug. They look for love to help them escape reality, to fix all their problems—to *save* them.

Boundaries have definitely been a challenge for me in some of my romantic relationships. I've been a serial monogamist for the past decade, jumping from one long-term relationship to the next. I have valued the comfort and safety of having another person to call my partner. I've also enjoyed the challenge of needing to make sacrifices to fulfill another person's needs for probably all the reasons I've mentioned above. It's given me a sense of purpose. It's made me feel safer in cases where my partner may have been somewhat dependent on me. And investing so much of my energy into worrying about someone else has served to distract me from my own problems and obligations.

In waking up to some of my patterns in romantic relationships, I am trying very hard to trust more (myself, my partner, and the universe) and to cling less to this idea that I need to be exactly who my partner needs me to be in every moment. I think making compromises for the person you love is a beautiful thing; it's certainly important to honor your partner's needs in addition to your own. It also deepens the bond between two people when both partners make an effort to show up for one another. However, it's also important that both partners trust and respect one another as individuals.

LIMIT EXPOSURE TO ENVIRONMENTS AND PERSONALITIES THAT DRAIN YOU

I recognize the kinds of environments that trigger negative feelings, make me feel uneasy, and drain my energy. Some examples of things that give me anxiety and deplete my energy—things I would call *energetically expensive*—include: crowded subway cars, loud parties, bars, clubs, Penn Station during rush hour, and grocery stores when they're overly crowded—with people competing for cart space in every aisle. Certain personality types deplete my energy as well. I tend to feel fatigued around people who are self-absorbed, people who are excessively extroverted, and people who need constant attention and validation, for example. People who are chronically pessimistic can be difficult to be around too.

On the other end of the spectrum, environments that restore my energy include being outside in nature, the silence and comfort of my own living space, comfortable coffee shops, bookstores, etc. And I feel invigorated when I am around people who are open-minded, kind, friendly, ambitious, and confident in themselves.

ALIGN YOUR EVERYDAY WORK WITH YOUR PERSONALITY

When I used to spend nearly nine hours a day, five days a week, bound to a computer for work, I'd be frustrated that I never had the time to write or play my guitar or try a new hobby like painting just for the hell of it. Never then had I considered that it wasn't about time, it was about *energy*. I was investing so much of my focused problem-solving energy into my job that I didn't have much left over at the end of the day to apply toward my own creative pursuits. Also, I'm not a person who really enjoys sitting still in the first place, so when I wasn't at work, the last thing I wanted to do was be stationary and focus my attention on another project—I wanted to go do something outside or do something physical. Because people generally spend more time working each week than anything else, this is a really important component of budgeting your energy—not giving it all to your job. I don't thrive in an office environment. Having to work under fluorescent lights and make frequent small talk throughout the day takes up a *lot* of my energy, whereas when I have the luxury of working from home, I am able to flow with my own productivity cycles each day, and I get more done in less time. Also, because I work mostly in isolation without much forced interaction throughout the day, I have an abundance of energy left over after work to put toward people and things that are important to me.

EXERCISE JUST ENOUGH BUT NOT TOO MUCH

Lastly, I find it important to be mindful of the way I spend my physical energy. As I divulged earlier, during my disordered days, I exercised obsessively, since I thought that amount of work was necessary to maintain a body I would feel comfortable in. I couldn't even conceive of the possibility that I could feel confident in my skin working out any less than six or seven days a week. But what I neglected to recognize then was the energetic deficit I experienced in other areas of my life due to prioritizing exercise to the extreme. The amount of actual time (not to mention mental space) it took each day to change into my gym clothes, commute to the gym, work out for an hour, commute home, make myself a smoothie, and shower left me with very little spare time or energy to invest in my relationships, hobbies, and passions. I have since experimented with different kinds of physical activity at different levels of intensity, frequency, and duration. I've found that I feel happiest when I work out three to four days a week for forty minutes to an hour. More than this feels like too much, and less doesn't provide me with the mental and physical benefits I need to feel good in my body.

When I exercise now, I enjoy it. I allow exercise to work for me rather than me working for it. When I'm craving nature, I go for a run or a bike ride outside. When I'm craving intensity, I take a kickboxing class. And when I'm stressed and my body feels out of alignment, I like doing yoga and other mindful activities. I no longer think of exercise as this rigid, inflexible thing, and I don't consider it at all without also considering how balance in this area will affect the balance in other areas of my life.

Chapter 12
Organize Your
Living Space to
Promote Wellbeing

-

Just as different environments and obligations
have an *energetic weight* to them, the items in your
physical space do too. Everything you choose to
make a part of your physical surroundings has the
power to make you feel either anxious or at peace.
Especially in this day and age, I think we have a
greater responsibility than prior generations to simplify
our lives in ways that protect our sanity. For example,
I make it a priority to routinely "weed out" some of
the excess in my life—that is, everything that takes up
room in my life without serving me on a practical or
spiritual level. This may include but is not limited to:
cleaning out my closet, deleting old emails, organizing
loose papers, and putting a limit on time spent with

technology and the amount of stimulation that enters my senses. This kind of routine maintenance is especially important in this modern age of information overload. With so much coming at us every minute of every day from so many angles, simplicity is not the default. It's something we need to work to cultivate for ourselves.

Marie Kondo, founder of the KonMari Method, wrote a great book on organization called *The Life-Changing Magic of Tidying Up: The Japanese Art of Decluttering and Organizing*. In the book, Kondo advocates for a more or less minimalist approach. While she provides plenty of specific and tangible methods for folding your clothing, organizing your closet, etc., the parts of the book I resonated with most were the principles behind the approach:

1. **Sort and purge by category, not by room.**

   It's best to pull out everything at once from a specific category (i.e., clothing, books, kitchen utensils). This way, you can assess the number of items you actually own that belong to this specific category. And when you sort through them, you'll probably have an easier time letting go of the "lowest ranking" items in each category, because you will be assessing them relative to items that you feel better about. For example, it will be easier to get rid of that old sweater that doesn't fit well when you see that you have five other sweaters you really like. And you can condense the number of pots and pans you own when you view the scratched-up ones next to those that are in better shape. This tends to be more effective than attacking one drawer or one room or one area at a time, in that most people's possessions are somewhat scattered rather than categorized by location.

2. **When determining whether to keep or discard an item, pick it up in your hands and focus on the way it makes you feel.**

This means relying more on your body for the answers than your mind, since our minds tend to make up excuses for items we own, such as, "Maybe I'll wear this if I lose ten pounds," or, "This is sentimental to me because I wore it when I met my girlfriend," or, "I may need this in case I go camping in the wilderness."

3. **Hold onto only what sparks joy and makes you feel happy.**

Since organizing my closet according to the KonMari method, it's been like a breath of fresh air each time I open my closet doors to get dressed in the morning. Every single item that has earned a hanger and its own piece of real estate is something I wear often and enjoy wearing. I've gotten rid of all my sentimental clothing and all my "conditional" clothing (for example, shirts I can only wear if I wear them under another shirt). The whole process of organizing my closet has helped me to get real with myself and embrace the present moment. Any item I feel resistant to wearing today, I am probably going to feel resistant to wearing tomorrow, too; so I let go of all the items that don't spark joy in the here and now.

4. Don't be sentimental.

This is not to say you shouldn't hold onto any sentimental possessions at all—keep the coins your deceased grandfather passed along to you, and keep the music box that's been passed down for five generations. But relieve yourself of anything you're holding onto purely because someone you love gave it to you: if it's not something that brings you joy, if it serves no practical purpose, and if it holds no significant value, then let go of it. This principle has been extremely useful me, since anything I had been hoarding had been for sentimental reasons—a gift from a friend or relative that I had never used or had grown out of, for example. Kondo offers an expert piece of advice to free emotional hoarders like myself from the confines of holding onto anything out of guilt. She suggests that anything you've received as a gift has already served its purpose, in that its purpose was to make you feel acknowledged and/or loved by the person who gave it to you. So essentially, all gifts fulfill their purpose in the moment they are received. By giving items away that no longer serve you, you set them free, and you set yourself free too. You can still go on loving the people that gave these gifts to you. In fact, when your living space is free of clutter, you'll be able to invest more of yourself into all your relationships and be capable of loving with fewer blockages. As a last resort, if you find you still have trouble letting go of a sentimental item that doesn't serve you, you can always take a picture of it! This usually takes up much less space than the actual thing. Then you are free to let the thing go.

5. Don't bury things in storage.

When you have fears and worries buried deep down in your subconscious, you may feel "stuck" in your life without knowing why. Similarly, if you have boxes and bins of stuff hidden away to the point that you don't even know what's there, you may feel burdened and out of control. Kondo suggests that nothing you own should really be put into storage. She even provides a folding method for "stacking" clothing in drawers so that no pieces of clothing are layered on top of other pieces of clothing—everything is visible. I have modified this rule just slightly for myself in that I do allow myself to store out of season clothing, backup drugstore items, and gym gear I don't use all that often. But these items are stored in neat bins that fit under my bed, where I can access them easily. Aside from what fits beneath my bed, nothing else I own is stored away.

I'll add to the list and say that in deciding which items I want to discard and which items I want to hold onto, I have found it helpful to consider the cost of living in New York City. Currently, I live in an apartment shared with two other people that costs $3,200 per month, not including utilities. To rent my room, about 154 square feet of living space, costs $1,100 per month. That means each square foot costs roughly $7.00 a month! So it's worth it for me to keep items that bring me joy and that I also use frequently, like my guitar and my skateboard. But the basketball I'll use maybe twice a year? Or the juicer under my bed I haven't used in over six months? Not worth the space. It would be more cost-effective for me to rent a basketball or borrow one from a friend if I ever want to play, and better for me to buy juice out at a juice place any time I feel like drinking some kale, even if they up the price a little.

Now you may be wondering by this point, why is all this information on organization inside a book on recovering from an eating disorder? But I swear to you that keeping a tidy living space is an absolutely essential part of self-care, and self-care is such an essential part of mental health. Especially for people recovering from eating disorders, it is essential to have a space of your own where you can feel comfortable, happy, safe, and at peace. I recommend also filling your space with fresh flowers, aromatherapy diffusers, candles, fresh fruit, and anything that makes you feel abundant and taken care of.

By simplifying, taming, and beautifying your space, you give yourself the opportunity to be exactly who you are in this moment. You free yourself from any baggage you've been holding onto from your past. You become more in touch with the person you are today and what you value, and less governed by former ideas of who or what you should be. And you make space—actual, tangible, physical space—for yourself to grow, evolve, and be.

Chapter 13
EAT MINDFULLY, BUT NOT NEUROTICALLY

-

"It is no measure of health to be well adjusted to a profoundly sick society."
—Jiddu Krishnamurti

-

Huddled around a New York City coffee truck, a group of stubbly-chinned men in construction hats gobble down donuts while talking and laughing in clouds of cigarette smoke. I can't help but observe them. What intrigues me about these men is that they have a carelessly comfortable way about them. Sure, they're killing themselves slowly with tobacco and sugar-laden breakfast pastries, yet somehow, they seem robustly healthy, authentically *real*. The men's faces are weathered, their jeans paint-stained and worn.

I imagine them to be ungoverned by hypothetical principles of wellbeing. They work to survive, they eat to get full, and their lives may be just that simple.

Moments later, I arrive at my very progressive, holistically conscious workplace for a meeting. The employees sit on Pilates balls instead of office chairs, and framed posters adorn the walls bearing phrases like, "Change your thoughts and you can change your world." Most of the nutritionally enlightened young people in the office drink green juice for breakfast or eat gluten-free toast with almond butter. By the hot water cooler, twenty-eight varieties of tea are stacked neatly in a wooden holder. Acknowledging the stark contrast between the diets and lifestyles I'd observed inside of thirty minutes' time, I think to myself, *Who's healthier? Who's happier? And what the hell am I supposed to eat in the modern world?*

The interesting challenge faced by former disordered eaters like myself is that you can't *end* your disorder with your bête noire, food, by simply cutting it out of your life. You're inevitably forced to make peace with it. An alcoholic knows what recovery looks like; recovery means no longer drinking. A drug addict knows, too, that to be clean means you're no longer using drugs. But to recover from an eating disorder, you must actually redefine your relationship with food. You have to transition from disordered eating to "normal" eating, and in order to do this, you must have a notion of "normal" eating to which to aspire.

Well, if you haven't noticed, the modern food climate in America is anything but normal. It's full of food that's fast, cheap, and processed, with no shortage of high fructose corn syrup, GMOs, artificial coloring, hormones, chemicals, and loads of other mystery ingredients. Produce grown with herbicides and pesticides is labeled "conventional," while produce grown without interference is labeled "organic." This kind of labeling implies that what's natural has become a specialized commodity, not something we're entitled to as our birthright. Our entire food chain has become vulnerable to this kind of corporate communism, not to mention the amount of animal cruelty and environmental pollution that are byproducts of the industry. Needless to say, it's become unfortunately necessary for people in the U.S. to apply a great deal of caution, education, and responsibility to making their food choices.

What's more, we are bombarded daily with all kinds of conflicting messages about what we should and shouldn't be consuming. One day, something's good for you, and the next, it causes cancer. One source tells you organic is worth the extra money, and another says produce is produce. You turn on the TV and see a commercial for a provocatively juicy whopper from Burger King followed by a Calvin Klein ad featuring "sexy" emaciated models. It's cruel and manipulative, this push-pull style of advertising that says "indulge, deprive, indulge, deprive," making a sport of people's attempts to live balanced lives. Given society's unrealistic expectations of consumers, it's no wonder that so many of us have developed unrealistic expectations of food.

If you've been relying solely on society, the food industry, and the media to tell you what to eat, by now you've been brainwashed to believe that you can't trust your body, your desires, or yourself. Perhaps you've bounced back and forth from one dieting extreme to another, stuck in a perpetual cycle of guilt, aspiration, and disillusionment. Or maybe you've rebelled as I did, in a silent battle against yourself. Especially for females in America, it can be difficult to trust our appetites in a culture that teaches us that merely having an appetite is *bad*. I swear to God, if I see one more yogurt commercial—they always show the same smiling, clear-skinned woman, savoring a spoonful from a single-serve container the size of baby food. Is this how women are supposed to spend their afternoons? Curled up in yoga pants on an oversized sofa, having an orgasm over a yogurt cup? One of Dannon's former slogans offended me so much that it's never left my mind: "Be light and fit. And satisfied," which in my mind translates to: "Eat the bare minimum to sustain life. And be okay with it."

Men, on the other hand, are marketed to in a way that's equally extreme, though it is taken in an extremely different direction. Let's take frozen dinners, for example. For women, you've got Lean Cuisine and Smart Ones. For men, it's Hungry Man Selects, with army stencil lettering and the slogan, "Eat like a man." What exactly does it mean to eat like a man? The way I read it is that the food industry assumes that as a man, your highest priorities are to be strong, large, and in charge. So men get Muscle Milk and aggressive product labels, while women get meek portions and pastel colors. I find the implications of such marketing campaigns to be oppressive to both sexes.

Nevertheless, women are the ones who suffer the brunt of it. We're the ones who walk away feeling as if our desires are in some way dirty or obscene. In fact, we're the only species on the planet taught to measure our self-worth by our ability to control our animal instincts. From the time we're very young, we are conditioned to believe that to be loved and accepted, we must control our hunger—break the bond of trust between body and mind. And for every pleasure, there must be repentance.

Perhaps this is why so many of us feel it's our duty to approach our diets with religious discipline. We've mistaken food for something of moral value, telling ourselves we are *good* if we eat this, and *bad* if we eat that (though no food is inherently sinful or righteous). We learn that to be successful, we must work hard, indulge sparingly, and control our impulses. God forbid we color outside the lines or live without parameters—bad things will happen if we let ourselves go.

So there's the food industry, corporate communism, and the media, which make it difficult for people to make sensible food choices to begin with. Then on top of this, many Americans just don't have a whole lot of room in their lives to devote to purchasing, preparing, and consuming healthy meals. Young people are working side jobs while going to school. Older people are working full-time along with caring for children and tending to life's other responsibilities. I'm a little embarrassed to admit this, but even working just thirty hours a week from home, I find myself having to be pretty strategic in order to maintain a work/life balance that affords me the time to take good care of myself. This includes: exercising, going grocery shopping for healthy ingredients, cooking healthy meals, cleaning up after myself, investing in relationships that fulfill me, spending time in nature, meditating, traveling to exciting places, and expanding into my creativity every once in a while. So I can't help but wonder—how are other people getting by? Well, the answer is that a lot of them *aren't* getting by. More people than ever before are suffering from anxiety, depression, insomnia, digestive issues, and fatigue. More are dying from nutrition and stress-related diseases. And more are addicted to pharmaceutical drugs.

Another factor contributing to what I'll refer to as "America's disorder" is that so many Americans have become segregated from nature in their modern-day lives. They rely on conflicting, disorienting, and illogical news and media sources to tell them what to do in terms of their own health. They hand off their bodies like foreign entities, entrusting them to the hands of doctors, hospitals, and drug companies. They've lost that sense of connectedness to something bigger.

In past ages, things were different. Our ancestors relied on nature for their survival, and so they interacted with it regularly and respected it deeply. People worked together in tribes and communities to hunt, gather, and harvest food; they were directly connected to the earth and its cycles. Contrast this with today's mile-a-minute society. Corporate communism and individualism have replaced tribes and togetherness. Children are not taught to appreciate the divinity of planting a seed and watching it grow—instead, they are glued to computers and other devices. Everything is outsourced and mass-produced. Convenience is at our fingertips, but we are over-accommodated in ways that strip us of our humanity and cause us to feel disconnected from everything we do.

Further, our senses are bombarded daily by social media, television, billboards, radios, newspapers, and magazines, not to mention the number of devices that beep, blink, and compete for our attention as technology claims more and more of our lives. Surrounded by so much noise and so many distractions, it can be a challenge to be able to hear the fragile voices within each of our souls. It's also energetically draining. I get decision fatigue just going to the grocery store when there are nineteen brands of toilet paper to choose from and seventeen different kinds of razors. I recognize that the freedom of having so many choices is part of what makes America "the land of the free." But I feel anything but liberated when faced with the responsibility of comparing twenty-six varieties of ketchup, requiring me to discern between twenty-six product labels and ingredient lists. It's no wonder so many people feel an emptiness inside, like an itch they just can't seem to scratch—their lives have been cluttered with excess and stripped of magic. They don't understand their purpose or their divinity because what they're yearning for may be something they've never even experienced before and therefore can't possibly imagine.

Now I'll return to my original question: what is *normal* when it comes to eating in modern times? To what extent are disorders to be seen as "disorders," and to what extent are they valid responses to a disordered world? While I consider myself fully recovered from my eating disorder insofar as I've come to heal on a spiritual and emotional level, there's still the reality of America's eating disorder to contend with, and the practical necessity of feeding myself well in a culture that tries very hard to misguide me.

Well, I certainly don't claim to have it all figured out, but the closest thing to balance I've been able to cultivate is this: I put as much time, energy, and money as I can afford into maintaining a healthy diet, but I don't let my diet cause me anxiety or rule my life. It is one part of my life, a part that's very important to me, but I don't let it steal my joy, compromise my freedom, or interfere with my relationships. I eat foods that are whole, natural, and local as often as possible. I eat consciously and intelligently with respect for the environment and other living beings, but I don't allow myself to become overly preoccupied with eating "perfectly." I'll drink green juice if I feel like it. I'll also eat pizza if I feel like it. At this point I know what works for my body and what satisfies me, and so it's become pretty much second nature for me to eat well without having to think about it too much or plan my life around it.

The way I eat now does not require any willpower. There's nothing I *should* consume and nothing I *shouldn't*. Rather, I choose to feed myself in a way that's healthy overall, because I value looking the way

I want to look and feeling the way I want to feel in my body. To be truly free, I believe, is to feed yourself in a way that considers every aspect of your evolving nature, and so I eat to nourish my cravings in the present while also setting myself up to feel good when I wake up tomorrow.

When operating from this mindset, it isn't difficult for me to say no to a chocolate donut or a bag of Doritos, because there is no internal conflict that pits *me* against *my body*. I am playing on my own team, not against myself. I *am* my body. On the other hand, I can also say yes to some junk food every now and then without being plagued with guilt afterwards. I trust myself to stop when I've had enough; I know my limits. I can eat until I'm satisfied using my intuition and maintain my ideal weight (I haven't weighed myself on a scale since I can remember, but I have worn the same clothing size for at least the past six years).

What it comes down to is trusting your body— when you decide to *integrate* your mind, your body, and your soul and work *with* nature, rather than against it, you no longer have to fight your cravings. Because when all parts of you are aligned, your cravings will not lead you to self-sabotage.

When I used to binge, it was often because I craved one simple thing that I refused to allow myself to consume, like a piece of chocolate, for example. Because I denied myself this reasonable amount of satiation, I would then spiral into a space where I lost all control. At first, I'd attempt to satisfy my sweet tooth with something "healthier" instead, like a bite of granola. But when granola didn't do the trick, I'd then reach for the next best substitute for chocolate, then the next. By the time I finally felt "satisfied," I'd have consumed way more calories than I would have had I just allowed myself the simple square of chocolate to begin with. The issue was that I pitted my mind against my body. I was so preoccupied with eating "correctly" that I let my mind do all the talking, never giving my body a chance to speak. And so my body rebelled by making its cravings known until they were satisfied.

If you find yourself binging, it's probably because you're overly restricting yourself the rest of the time. I can tell you from experience that when you stop restricting and depriving yourself, you will stop obsessing and binging and abusing food. We're all animals, after all. And if you force any animal into a period of famine, it's going to trigger a primal survival mechanism which will make that animal eat uncontrollably once a food source becomes available again. You can't fight nature and win. Remember that.

All right, so I've told you where I'm at these days when it comes to food—now let me tell you how I got here. It certainly wasn't an overnight kind of thing. I struggled for a while. For years I told myself I was "recovered" because I had stopped starving myself and stopped throwing up. But during those years, I was still preoccupied with food in ways that led me to constantly experiment with it to gain perspective. I went on a few different "health" fasts. I tried going raw, vegan, and vegetarian, all for short periods of time. I tried eliminating sugar, gluten, dairy, and soy, and I observed the way I felt under each new set of restrictions. I probably fit the criteria for orthorexia during this time, which is a condition that includes symptoms of obsessive behavior in pursuit of a healthy diet. A person with orthorexia is obsessed with defining and maintaining the "perfect" diet, rather than an ideal weight.[6] They tend to fixate on their own personal definition of "righteous eating," which usually includes eating foods they believe to be pure,

---

6. Timberline Knolls Residential Treatment Center. "Orthorexia Symptoms and Effects." http://www.timberlineknolls.com/eating-disorder/orthorexia/signs-effects/ (accessed 2017).

healthy, and of a certain quality, while avoiding foods they believe to be unclean or unworthy.

I went on this way for a while, convincing myself I was taking care of myself—convincing myself my still-neurotic behaviors were coming from self-love—until the day I woke up and realized my love for myself would be truer if I permitted myself to give less of a fuck. I don't have to be super disciplined to be healthy. I don't have to sacrifice flavor or pleasure to feel confident in my skin. I just have to make decisions for myself that are rooted in love rather than fear. Yes, it's necessary to be educated and proactive in order to eat reasonably well in America. And yet, I was tired of the hours of food preparation and mixing green powders that tasted like grass into all of my beverages and taking it to the extreme. Although I had been eating a diet that consisted almost entirely of natural food, the amount of effort and discipline it took to maintain it felt completely unnatural. It was then that I became determined to find a way to incorporate healthy eating into my life without it requiring all my energy. So slowly but surely, I started incorporating more diversity into my diet. ("If I eat an organic green salad with chicken for lunch, can I permit myself to order takeout for dinner? Sure!") I also started taking more shortcuts, like buying produce that's pre-chopped and buying frozen rice that's pre-cooked, even if it costs a little bit more, because I value my time.

Julia Child once said, "People who love to eat are always the best people," and I think there's a lot of truth to this. In being able to welcome food into our lives with a relaxed affection that is free of shame, we welcome other forms of nourishment into our lives with the same energy of openness. We empower ourselves and the people around us to expand on a heart level. I believe that regardless of what we actually eat, if we're filling ourselves with love and sharing that love with others, we are going to make the planet more sustainable for us all. Calories, after all, are a measure of *energy*, and everything we eat as well as everything we do has the power to nourish or deplete us.

Today, I feel more at peace with food than I have in my entire life, and I'm tempted to say it's *because* I've been to hell and back with it. I've struggled, experimented, and explored food with so much patience and curiosity over time that I've found a way to coexist with it gracefully. I've learned to read my body's fine print, and I believe anyone is capable of doing the same.

It's extremely rare these days for me to feel any sense of guilt around eating, but should the feeling arise, I take it as a cue that there's something deeper going on in my body that I need to pay attention to. I communicate with myself rather than escaping through extreme thought patterns and extreme dieting.

In the end, eating well isn't about being a slave to your diet or enduring feelings of anxiousness, apprehension, and isolation just to maintain a diet that's "clean." It's living in harmony with food, the environment, other people, and most importantly, yourself. It's surrendering control, not hoarding it. It's respecting nature and tuning in to the sacred intuition that lives inside us all.

If you are in the process of healing from an eating disorder or other addiction, my advice to you is to be kind to yourself and be patient. Balance is a journey, not a destination. Just as a gymnast must find her center with each step she takes along a balance beam, we're all continuously evolving, and therefore we must remain mindful and willing to continuously adjust ourselves. At the end of the day, there is no right or wrong way to nourish yourself; there's only the amount of awareness, responsibility, and love you choose to bring to the table.

Chapter 14
CHECK IN WITH YOURSELF
AS YOU EVOLVE

-

Get to know yourself so that you can nurture your unique needs and show up to your life every day as your best self. But it's also important to check in with yourself as you evolve. Don't limit yourself by clinging to various lists of criteria and ideas about who you are. Instead, embrace the freedom to experience yourself every day without preconceived notions. In every new moment, you have the opportunity to surprise yourself, reinvent yourself, act spontaneously, and try new things.

It can be liberating in the process of cultivating self-awareness to create certain labels for yourself that help define you for others, so that you feel accepted as part of a community. However, just because you consider yourself to be something one day doesn't mean you will resonate with that forever. I'd always considered myself to be an introvert, for example, and I still am in that I still require alone time to recharge. However, since I have gotten to know myself better and come to love myself, I am a whole lot more social than I used to be, and it opens me up in many ways to acknowledge that. My tolerance for being around other people for long periods of time without feeling depleted has doubled, if not tripled, from what it used to be. I even crave the company of others much of the time.

I think a lot of people make the mistake of labeling experiences as failures just because those experiences don't pan out the way they expected. Couples fall in love and get married only to find themselves growing apart years later as they both evolve, and at that point they may separate. But this doesn't have to be viewed as a "failed" marriage. It can instead be viewed as a successful marriage that didn't last forever. A person might begin to pursue a particular career path only to decide later, after learning more about the field (and learning more about themselves), that it isn't a fit. Such is life.

Nothing is static and nothing is guaranteed. But also, the end doesn't always justify the means. Sometimes we all have to take certain risks or make certain commitments in order to get to know ourselves better. And just because an experience lasts for a period of time rather than forever doesn't indicate failure and doesn't mean the experience didn't contribute value and meaning to your life.

I'll share with you a personal example relating to my sexuality. I started defining myself as a lesbian from around the age of eighteen, when I first discovered I was attracted to women, and I clung very fiercely to this label for many years. However, more recently, I've begun to identify more with the term queer, which is more like a state of mind than a sexual orientation. So I'm thirty-one years old, and I'm committing to a new word to explain my sexuality, and I'm embracing it— because what's the point of living if you don't live with an open heart and allow yourself to be affected by new possibilities that enter your senses as you continuously rediscover yourself?

I'm going to share with you the following article from the *Huffington Post* because it ties together a lot of the perspectives I've discussed in this book, in addition to being something I resonate with on a very deep level:

Being Queer Means...
By Nadia Cho

"Queer" is not a term that is universally recognized and understood in the common vernacular. So I will attempt to present the many different sides of what being queer means. "Queer" can be used to describe someone's sexual orientation or stand as a political statement. Its definition has many dimensions, from gender identification to a resistance against structural rigidity to a strange sensation or state of being. "Queer" isn't a word that many people clearly understand when used to describe yourself. Allow me to elaborate what being queer personally means to me, as "queer" means different things to different people.

Being queer is first and foremost a state of mind. It is a worldview characterized by acceptance, through which one embraces and validates all the unique, unconventional ways that individuals express themselves, particularly with respect to gender and sexual orientation. It is about acknowledging the infinite number of complex, fluid identities that exist outside the few limited, dualistic categories considered legitimate by society. Being queer means believing that everyone has the right to be themselves and express themselves without being judged or hated because that doesn't fit in with what's normal. Being queer means challenging everything that's considered normal.

Being queer means ceasing to think in binaries like "male" or "female," "gay" or "straight," "monogamous" or "non-monogamous," because there are more than two sides to every person and every context. It means being aware of and OK with the fact that our own identities and sexualities are always in flux, never static. Being queer means recognizing that there are alternate gender identities, such as transgender or genderqueer or androgynous folks, and respecting that these identities are just as legitimate as those that are visible.

A queer worldview deconstructs and obliterates all established notions of gender. Gender is a set of socially constructed roles arbitrarily assigned to everyone based on physiological reproductive traits. Being queer means embracing supposedly "masculine" and "feminine" traits as simply universal human traits and ignoring the behavioral expectations that are socially imposed according to our non-consensually assigned gender. Genitals don't tell men that they can't wear dresses and women that they have to wait to be asked out; cultural norms dictate gendered behaviors. Being queer means doing away with gender altogether, because it restricts the ways people can freely and unlimitedly express themselves.

Being queer means being attracted to anyone, with no regard to a person's gender or sex. It could mean someone is attracted to more than one gender, or even two genders. Being queer means you like what you like and you accept that your desires are dynamic and you are open to change. Being queer means being sex-positive and recognizing that sex is good and everyone has the right to have as much or as little of it as suits them. It means thinking about sex in different ways other than the heterosexual, male-pleasure-oriented, meant-for-reproduction kind.

Being queer means constantly questioning what's considered "normal" and why that norm gets privileged over other ways of being. It means criticizing who sets these norms and recognizing the privilege that comes with being able to identify as "normal." Being queer means confronting all forms of oppression and bringing unheard minority experiences and stories to light. Being queer means addressing and understanding the intersectionality between race, gender, sexuality, and class and how it affects each person's experience and identity differently.

Being queer means searching for alternate ways of being and living. It means learning to appreciate and celebrate difference and striving for constructive, fair and happy ways to coexist with each other. Being queer means constantly looking for ways to be as inclusive as possible in order to create a world where everyone feels safe and accepted, in which there is true equality for every single person.

Being queer means embracing a free and open-ended identity by casting off all other identities that categorize us, and defining ourselves simply as human beings.[7]

---

7. Cho, Nadia. "Being Queer Means...." Huffington Post. https://www. huffingtonpost.com/nadia-cho/being-queer-means_b_3510828.html (accessed 2017).

I am going to go out on a limb here and say
I think the world could benefit from more people
adopting a queer mindset and accepting that ideas and
identities are fluid rather than fixed. Regardless of who
or what you choose to have sex with, let's leave that
part out of it and focus on the beauty that can come
from seeing others and ourselves as transient beings in
transient states of being.

Here's some advice straight from me to you: take
risks, aspire to achieve new goals, take action steps
toward trying out the thing you are most curious
about, meet new people, be curious, ask questions,
and breathe new light into each new day. Adjust
the way you navigate your life based on everything
that comes your way. Make the time to check in and
explore yourself on a regular basis.

Chapter 15
Final Words

-

"Life isn't about waiting for the storm to pass...it's about learning to dance in the rain."
–Vivian Greene

-

There is a nineteen-year-old girl still alive in my mind. I can feel her fragile body standing upon my heart, the imprints of her feet as she weighs herself against an infinity of things she doesn't feel she measures up to. I watch her stare into the mirror as she holds up her shirt and studies the way her stomach caves inward. I can see the spaces between her ribs and the form of her pelvis, a butterfly made of bone, unable to fly. If I could only transcend the barrier of time, I'd go back and kneel down beside this girl. I'd grab her cold hands and tell her she's already enough. I'd tell her that everything will get better, *trust me*.

The way I see it now, suffering is not always the same as pain. Sometimes suffering is a choice that comes from *avoiding* pain, or avoiding life. Anyone can self-destruct. Self-destructing is easy. It neglects to ask questions. Like a toxic parasite, self-destruction cares only about being fed. It doesn't care who you are or what you need. Self-love, on the other hand, is all about curiosity and asking questions. When you love yourself, you check in with yourself frequently. You pay attention to all the things that have the ability to nourish or deplete you, and you make choices that are productive rather than destructive to your wellbeing.

I respect my body now the way I respect the ocean—I know there are miles of wisdom and mystery below the surface that remain undiscovered. I think of every year, every month, every day, and every second I have been alive, and I know there's a brilliance my body holds by which I can be guided, whether or not I comprehend it entirely. There is so much available to me, as long as I'm willing to inhabit my body for long enough to hear what it's saying.

The process of coming to love myself has been an art, not a science. It's taken courage, patience, experimentation, and having compassion for myself throughout it all. I will never be the master of my own life, just as you will never be the master of yours. But I will embrace my life as a beautiful gift; I will let it bloom. I'll acknowledge that there is so much value in taking responsibility for the things for which I *can* take responsibility. And there is so much beauty in surrendering to the rest.

I'd go as far as to say that in cultivating the ability to tolerate uncertainty, we might even approach death with less resistance. We are all going to die one day. This is a lesson nature teaches us over and over again—the leaves change color in autumn and fall to the ground, relationships lessen in intensity and end, and loved ones pass away. No matter how good you are at convincing yourself you're in control along the way, birth and death are the only two experiences that are guaranteed to every human being. Sometimes we need to confront the silence, or even our own mortality and the impermanence of all things, in order to bring ourselves peace and freedom while we are alive.

As human individuals in modern times, every one of us has a tremendous responsibility to live authentically in a world that's polluted with so many influential forces. We all have the opportunity to broaden our realities and expand our culture to include new options and possibilities for everyone, rather than asking people to change themselves to fit into boxes and standardized molds and outdated expectations. And I think it's really necessary that we make this a priority.

There is all this dogma out there that says, "Be a good person." But you know what? It's not about being a *good* person. It's about being a truthful person. When you live in a way that's true to you and the people around you, and when you feel free and happy in your skin, you will be "good" as a consequence. You will treat people kindly, you'll inspire them effortlessly, and you will spread joy to those who need it the most.

When I think of the notion of God, I don't look up. I look around me. I finally understand what it means to be present—it's existing in a state of gratitude and trust, rather than of expectation and disillusionment. Everything there is to seize and appreciate is right here, right now. For me, just feeling connected to this divinity is enough to eliminate my need to control it.

Reader, if I can leave you with one thing, I encourage you to follow your curiosity with the best intentions and forgive yourself when things don't go according to plan. When you forgive yourself, you give yourself permission to be human. And human is what you are. So let go and trust the mystery. Release the expectation that you should have total control over your life's circumstances. Enlightenment is not having the discipline to escape our bodies; it's having the courage to be present within them.

Additional Resources

In addition to the topics in this book and my suggestions for recovery, I want to emphasize the importance of seeking professional support if you are in an acute stage of an eating disorder or struggling with your identity or sexuality.

Below is a list of beginner-level resources I have compiled. Some are national and some are New York-based. I encourage you to search online to locate current support groups, counselors, therapists, and other resources in your local area.

EATING DISORDER RESOURCES

The National Eating Disorders Association
nationaleatingdisorders.org

NEDA supports individuals and families affected by eating disorders, and serves as a catalyst for prevention, research into cures, and access to quality care.

The National Association of Anorexia Nervosa and Associated Disorders
anad.org

ANAD is a nonprofit organization which assists people struggling with eating disorders and provides resources, support, and education for families, schools, and the eating disorder community.

The Alliance for Eating Disorders Awareness

allianceforeatingdisorders.com

The Alliance is a nonprofit organization dedicated to providing programs and activities aimed at outreach, education, and early intervention for all eating disorders.

Academy for Eating Disorders (AED)

aedweb.org

The Academy for Eating Disorders is a global professional association committed to leadership in eating disorders, research, education, treatment, and prevention.

Binge Eating Disorder Association (BEDA)

bedaonline.com

The Binge Eating Disorder Association is the national organization focused on providing leadership in the recognition, prevention, and treatment of Binge Eating Disorder (BED).

Eating Disorder Hope

eatingdisorderhope.com

Eating Disorder Hope offers education, support, and inspiration to eating disorder sufferers, their loved ones, and eating disorder treatment providers.

Anorexia Nervosa and Related Eating Disorders (ANRED)

anred.com

ANRED is a website dedicated to making it easier for people to learn about eating disorders and how to recover from them.

Monte Nido: Eating Disorder Treatment Center

montenido.com

Monte Nido is a residential treatment center for eating disorders with several locations around the United States.

The Freedom Institute

freedominstitute.org

Freedom Institute is a New York State OASAS licensed, medically supervised outpatient addiction treatment services and recovery center located in midtown Manhattan.

Chelsea Roff | Eat Breathe Thrive

chelsearoff.com

eatbreathethrive.org

Eat Breath Thrive is a nonprofit organization that aims to prevent and help individuals overcome food and body image challenges through integrative mind-body programs.

To Write Love on Her Arms (TWLOHA)

twloha.com

To Write Love on Her Arms is a nonprofit movement dedicated to providing hope and finding help for people struggling with depression, addiction, self-injury, and suicide.

Geneen Roth

geneenroth.com

Geneen Roth is the author of the #1 *New York Times* bestseller *Women Food and God.* She is a writer and teacher whose work focuses on using addiction as a path to the inner universe.

Eating Disorders Coalition

eatingdisorderscoalition.org

The EDC advances the recognition of eating disorders as a public health priority throughout the United States.

SEXUALITY AND IDENTITY RESOURCES

The Trevor Project

thetrevorproject.org

The Trevor Project is the leading national organization providing crisis intervention and suicide prevention services to LGBTQ young people ages thirteen to twenty-four.

The Center | The Lesbian, Gay, Bisexual & Transgender Community Center

gaycenter.org

The Center is a New York City-based environment offering the LGBT communities of NYC health and wellness programs; arts, entertainment and cultural events; recovery, wellness, parenthood and family support services.

IHI Therapy Center

ihitherapy.com

IHI is a NYC-based nonprofit psychotherapy and training center dedicated to fostering personal growth free of traditional gender, sexual orientation, and cultural biases.

Notes

Notes

Notes

Notes

Notes

Notes

Notes

Notes

Notes

Notes

Acknowledgments

Thank you to my sister, Kristy. You read the earliest drafts of *Starving in Search of Me* when it was only beginning to take shape and felt heavy and opaque. Knowing I was going to receive your feedback kept me motivated during the most grueling hours I spent writing in solitude, before anyone else was involved in bringing this to fruition. Your involvement has been most valuable since you share many of my experiences and could provide an objective yet very connected perspective.

Thank you to my parents, Lenny and Ginny. Since I was a child, you have encouraged, supported, and celebrated all of my creative endeavors. You've provided me confidence and safety in who I am, inspiring me to embrace my independence, travel down the longest roads, and reach for the stars. And you've happily and proudly spread the word about my book to everyone you know.

Thank you to my girlfriend, Yasmin. You made me laugh and helped me to reconnect with my playful spirit during the final tedious year I spent stuck in my head, refining my manuscript. You've been supportive of my book every step of the way, even when it meant sitting with me for hours in cafés on weekends so that I could meet my deadlines.

Thank you to my agent, Ellen White. You agreed to represent my book because you fell in love with the writing. You saw me, you trusted me, and you gave me a chance based on my potential and your intuition, even before I put any work into anything more than the words on the page. Thank you also for having my back throughout the process, and for remaining emotionally connected to my vision throughout.

Thank you to Mango Publishing for investing in books by progressive authors whose voices the world needs to hear. The day we signed a contract together, everything finally made sense. There is no feeling comparable to finally being recognized after pouring your heart and soul into something for years with no guarantee. Thank you also for your support, and for holding me accountable.

Thank you to Amanda Filippelli for professionally editing earlier versions of *Starving in Search of Me*, and for helping me to find its heart and structure when it had no spine.

Thank you to Lindsey Smith for generously supporting my work and for being a friend and mentor to me when it comes to all things related to writing, publishing, and marketing a book.

And thank you to my community of friends and followers. Without your support, engagement, and encouragement, I would not be nearly as motivated.

About the Author

Marissa LaRocca is an award-winning New York-based writer, speaker, and activist. She is passionate about helping adolescents and young women embrace their individuality and overcome challenges related to emotional eating, self-acceptance, identity, sexuality, body image, and depression. She is on a mission to help others with her activism.

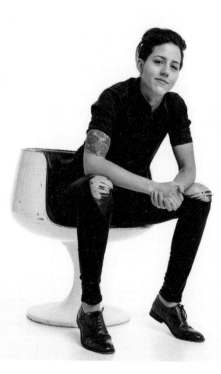